MW01236019

GLUTEN-FREE BREAD MACHINE RECIPE BOOK

A Collection of 122 Easy Gluten-Free Bread Machine Recipes to Satisfy Your Cravings [A Cookbook]

Author: Ashley Winebarger

Table of Content

Introduction: 5

What is Gluten-Free Bread? 7

BREAKFAST BREAD **8**

1. Banana Bread 8

2. Maple Oat Bread 9

3. Pear Cake Bread 10

4. Carrot Cake 11

5. Maple Bread 12

5. Chickpea Bread 13

7. Oat Bread 14

8. Potato Bread with Ricotta Cheese 15

9. Sourdough White Bread 16

10. Low-Carb Bread 17

11. Mediterranean Bread 18

12. Paleo Bread 19

13. Cinnamon, Fruit, and Raisin Bread 20

BASIC GLUTEN-FREE BREAD **21**

14. White Bread 21

15. Brown Bread 22

16. Multigrain Bread 23

17. Sorghum Bread 24

18. Barley Bread 25

19. High Protein Gluten Free Bread 26

20. Oat & Rice Bread 27

21. Sourdough Bread 29

22. Yeast-Based Paleo Bread 30

23. Wholemeal Bread 31

SWEET BREAD **33**

24. Cinnamon Raisin Bread 33

25. Apple Spice Bread 34

26. Cherry Bread 35

27. Hawaiian Sweet Bread 36

28. Autumn Pumpkin Bread 37

29. Zucchinni Bread 38

30. Banana and hemp bread 39

31. Bread Recipe Without Flaxseed Meal 40

32. Green Tea Bread 41

33. Brioche Bread 42

34. Butter Pecan Supreme Bread 43

SAVORY BREAD **44**

35. Sun Dried Tomato Bread 44

36. Jalapeno Corn Bread 45

37. Herb & Olive Loaf Bread 46

38. Onion Bread 47

39. Cheddar Cheese Bread 48

40. Garlic Parmesan Bread 49

41. Nut Freratae Low-Carb Bread 50

42. Cheese Loaf Bread 51

43. Pumpernickel Bread 52

44. Rye Bread 54

45. Potato Bread 55

46. Black Russian Bread 56

47. Lemon Cheesecake 57

48. Bread Recipe with Cacao and Fennel 59

PIZZA AND SANDWICH **60**

49. Pizza Dough 60

50. Smoked Salmon Salad Pizza 62

51. Pizza Crust 64

52. Pizza Recipe 65

53. Sandwich Bread 66

54. Sorghum-Millet Sandwich Bread 67

55. Sandwich Bread and Dinner Rolls 68

56. Halloween Sandwich Cookies 70

57. Polenta with Mushrooms 71

58. Multi-Grain Sandwich Bread 72

59. Rosemary Sandwich Bread 73

QUICK BREAD **74**

60. Corn Bread 74

61. No Yeast Bread 75

62. Beer Bread 77

63. Bread with Bacon & Olives 79

64. Sweet Potato Cornbread with Walnuts 80

65. Sourdough Onion Bread with Pumpkin 81

66. Baguettes Recipe 82

67. Cranberry, Pumpkin & Pecan Bread 83

68. Sourdough Rye Bread 84

69. Apple Walnuts Cake 85

70. Artisan Bread 86

71. Light Mock Rye Bread 87

NUTS & SEEDS BREAD **88**

72. Nuts and Seeds Bread 88

73. Seed Bread 89

74. Oatnut 3-Seed Bread 90

75. Goji Berries Bread 92

76. Christmas Nut Bread 93

77. Chestnut & Rice Flour Bread 94

78. Walnut Honey Bread 95

79. Molasses Walnut Bread 96

80. Date Nut Bread 97

81. Sunflower Seed Bread 98

82. Seeded Brown Bread 99

83. Flaxseed Bread 100

84. Linseed Brown Bread 101

85. Brown Rice Millet Bread 102

86. Psyllium Husk Bread 103

VEGETARIAN BREAD 104

87. French Bread 104

88. Vegan Bread 105

89. Italian Herb Bread 106

90. Rice Flour & Buckwheat Bread 107

91. Sesame Bread 108

92. Pumpkin Bread 109

93. Vegan Cinnamon Raisin Bread 110

94. Garlic Bread 111

95. Banana Bread with Pumpkin 112

96. Brown Rice Vegan Bread 113

97. Quinoa Chickpea Vegan Bread 114

98. Brown Rice Bread 115

99. Cassava Century Bread 116

100. Cocont Flour Bread 117

101. Brown Rice and Cranberry Bread 118

102. Millet Chia Bread 119

103. Buckwheat Bread 120

104. Buttermilk Bread 121

105. Brown and White Bread 122

106. Salt Free White Rice Bread 123

107. Hamburger Buns 125

108. Pear and Chocolate Galette 126

109. Brioche Burger Buns 127

110. Dairy-Free Dinner Rolls 128

111. Soft Dinner Roll 129

112. Cinnamon Rolls 130

FRUIT BREAD 131

113. Cinnamon Fruit and Seed Loaf 131

114. Dried Fruits Bread 132

115. Fruit Loaf 133

116. Fruit Bread 134

117. Fruit Pecan Bread 135

118. Festive Fruit Bread 136

119. Cardamom Flavored Fruit Bread 137

120. Toasted Oat Fruit Bread 138

121. Ripe Banana Bread 139

122. Bread with Sundried Tomatoes and Parmesan 140

INTRODUCTION:

Welcome to the "Gluten-Free Bread Machine Recipe Book," your passport to a world where delicious, warm, home-baked bread and a gluten-free lifestyle not only coexist but harmonize beautifully!

For so many, bread is more than food - it's a cherished ritual, a comfort, a daily staple. So when faced with a gluten-free diet, for whatever reason, you may feel you're bidding farewell to the joy of baking and savoring these delightful loaves. But let's debunk that myth right here and now. The world of gluten-free bread is just as vast, just as tantalizing, and brimming with a stunning variety of textures and flavors. Yes, there's absolutely no reason to compromise on your love for bread.

This book will help you to explore and learn and master gluten-free baking. It will be great for experienced bakers who want to try gluten-free baking for the first time and also for people who are just starting to make bread for the first time in general. It's designed to make the process fun, easy, and satisfying, ensuring you can enjoy your journey in the culinary world without the worry of gluten.

We've carefully curated recipes that blend traditional bread-making methods with a modern, health-conscious approach. You'll find dozens of delicious, creative recipes—from rustic whole grain loaves to sweet, decadent dessert bread—all crafted to taste great and be kind to your digestive system. Each recipe is tailored for your bread machine, transforming it into a magical gluten-free bakery at your fingertips.

But it's not just about the recipes. We'll take you on an adventure through the nuances of gluten-free grains, flours, and ingredients, arming you with the knowledge to adapt recipes or even create your own. You'll become a gluten-free gourmet, understanding how to mix and match flavors, how to get the right texture, and most importantly, how to make bread that everyone—gluten-free or not—will love.

Our promise to you is simple: with this book in your kitchen, you'll never miss gluten again. So let's warm up the bread machine, dust off your apron, and get ready to embark on an incredible gluten-free adventure, one loaf at a time. Your taste buds are in for an unforgotten treat! Welcome to the wonderful world of gluten-free bread machine baking!

GLUTEN FREE BREAD MACHINE RECIPE BOOK

BASIC GLUTEN-FREE BREAD

BREAKFAST BREAD

SWEET BREAD

QUICK BREAD

FRUIT BREAD

SAVORY BREAD

PIZZA AND SANDWICH

NUTS & SEEDS BREAD

VEGETARIAN BREAD

WHAT IS GLUTEN-FREE BREAD?

Gluten-free bread is a type of bread that does not contain gluten, a protein which found in wheat, barley, rye, and their derivatives. Gluten provides elasticity and structure to bread and helps it rise during baking. However, individuals with celiac disease, gluten intolerance, or gluten sensitivity need to avoid gluten-containing foods, including regular bread, as they can cause various adverse reactions.

Gluten-free bread is made using alternative grains and flour that do not contain gluten, such as rice, corn, soy, tapioca, or potato. When mixed with gluten-free binders like xanthan gum or guar gum, these ingredients help gluten-free bread have the same texture and structure as regular bread.

Gluten-free bread can be found in various forms, including sliced bread, rolls, baguettes, and other specialty bread products. While it aims to resemble regular bread, it may have a slightly different texture, taste, and appearance due to the absence of gluten. Manufacturers often use additional ingredients, such as eggs, milk, or honey, to enhance the flavor and texture of gluten-free bread.

It's important to note that not all gluten-free bread is suitable for individuals with celiac disease or severe gluten intolerance, as cross-contamination can occur during production or handling. To ensure safety, individuals with such conditions should look for certified gluten-free products and carefully read ingredient labels for any potential sources of gluten.

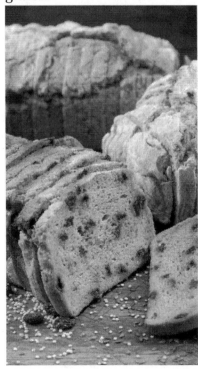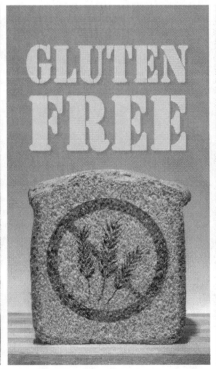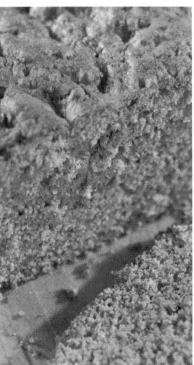

1. BANANA BREAD

Prep Time: 15 Minutes

Cooling Time: 1 hour

Cook Time: 1 hour

Total Times: 2 hours 15 Minutes

Serving: 8-10

Ingredients

- 1 cup of sugar
- 1 1/2 tsp. baking powder
- 1/2 cup of butter, melted
- 1/2 tsp. salt
- 2 eggs, beaten
- 1/4 cup of sour cream
- 1/2 cup of pecans, chopped

- 1 tsp. vanilla extract
- 1/3 cup of milk
- 2 cups of all-purpose flour
- 1 tsp. baking soda
- 3 medium-sized bananas, very ripe (or frozen and thawed), mashed

Instructions

1. Pour all of the ingredients in the order listed into the bread pan. Set the machine to the setting for quick bread with a medium crust and turn it on.
2. If the top of the bread still doesn't look done, leave it in the bread machine while it's still warm for 10 minutes or until it's done.
3. After 10 minutes, take the loaf out of the pan using oven mitts because it will still be hot. Remove the mixing paddle from the bottom of the loaf as well.
4. Let the bread cool all the way down on a wire rack. Cut it up and serve.

2. MAPLE OAT BREAD

Prep Time: 10 Minutes | Cook Time: 1 hour 20 Minutes

Total Times: 3 hours 30 Minutes | Serving: 12 Slice

Ingredients

- 1/3 cup of pure maple syrup
- 3/4 cup of + 1 tbsp non-fat milk (or water for dairy-free)
- 1/4 cup of neutral-flavored oil (6 tbsp using sorghum flour)
- 1 tsp of gluten-free apple cider vinegar
- 3 large eggs at room temperature
- 1-1/2 cups of certified gluten-free oat flour
- 1/2 cup of cornstarch
- 1 cup of + 2 tbsp potato starch
- 1 tbsp xanthan gum
- 2-1/4 tsp instant dry yeast
- 1-1/2 to 2 tsp seeds of choice
- 1 tsp oats or seeds for topping(optional)
- 2 tsp gluten-free oats or seeds for mixing in (optional)
- 1 tsp salt (optional)

Instructions

1. To bake in a Bread Machine with a Gluten-Free Setting:
2. Take the pan out of the bread maker. Check to make sure the paddle is attached.
3. Put the milk or water, maple syrup, oil, vinegar, and eggs in the bread machine's bowl.
4. Whisk the oat flour, potato starch, cornstarch, xanthan gum, yeast, salt, and seeds, if using, together in a separate bowl. Put into the bread machine's bowl.
5. Put the bowl in the machine with a snap. Choose the gluten-free option from the menu on your machine and press "Start."Place a silicone or rubber spatula, and scrape the flour from the pan's sides during the 1st few minutes of the mixing cycle.
6. When the mixing is done, take the mixing paddle out. Take your spatula to smooth out the top.
7. If you want to put oats or seeds on top of your bread, add them now and press them in with the backs of your wet fingers.
8. When the baking cycle is done, use the loaf out of the pan and take it on a wire rack to cool for 1.5 to 2 hours.
9. Once it has cooled, use a steak knife to take out the paddle.
10. Use an electric slicer, an electric knife, or a serrated knife to cut the bread. Even though you can leave the bread out on the counter overnight, the best way to store gluten-free bread is to cut it up and freeze it. Then reheat in the microwave, or heat a wet paper towel in the microwave and wrap the bread in it until it's defrosted.

3. PEAR CAKE BREAD

Prep Time: 20 Minutes | Cook Time: 2-3 Minutes

Total Times: 2 hours 20 Minutes - 3 Hours 20 Minutes

Serving: 1 Slice

Ingredients

- 3 eggs
- 2 tsp of vanilla extract
- 3 cups of gluten-free all-purpose flour
- 2 cups of white sugar
- 1 tsp of salt
- ¾ cup of vegetable oil
- 1 tsp of baking powder
- ¼ tsp of baking soda
- 2 cups of peeled and shredded pears
- 1 tbsp of ground cinnamon

Instructions

1. Put everything in the bread pan in the order specified in the recipe, then choose the gluten-free, 2-pound loaf with a medium crust setting. If you cut the amount of ingredients to fit the settings on your machine, make the necessary changes.
2. Take the pecans to the dough mixture when the machine beeps to add nuts. The moment the bread has risen in the machine put the thin slices of pear on top and close the lid quickly.
3. When the loaf is done, let it sit for 10 minutes, then put it out of the pan and let it on a wire rack to cool.

4. CARROT CAKE

Prep Time: 20 Minutes | Cook Time: 30 Minutes

Total Times: 55 Minutes | Serving: 10 Slice

Ingredients

- 2/3 cup of (79.3g) white sorghum flour
- 1/3 cup of (46.7g) potato starch
- 2/3 cup of (144g) olive oil
- 1 cup of (148g) brown rice flour
- 1 tsp. (2.1g) ground nutmeg
- 1 tsp. (2.5g) xanthan gum
- 1 cup of (198g) sugar
- 4 Tbsp. (58.8g) apple sauce

- 2 Tbsp. (13.0g) flaxseed meal
- 1 tsp. (5.3g) baking soda
- 3 Tbsp. (42.0g) hot water (195°F-208°F)
- 1 tsp. (2.0g) ground cinnamon
- 1-1/8 cup of (124.5g) peeled and shredded carrot
- 3 Tbsp. (21.0g) tapioca flour
- 5 tsp. (17.5g) baking powder

Instructions

1. Put the flaxseed meal and hot water in a bowl and let it stay for around 10 minutes.
2. Mix the flour ingredients (white sorghum flour, brown rice flour, potato starch, tapioca flour, xanthan gum, baking powder, baking soda, ground cinnamon, and ground nutmeg) and sugar well with a whisk in a large bowl.
3. With a whisk, mix the flaxseed meal solution, apple sauce, and olive oil well in a separate bowl. Add the carrot shreds. Make sure the kneading blade(s) are attached correctly and then pour the dough into the baking pan.
4. Pour the flour mixture into the baking pan.
5. Put the baking pan in the Home Bakery, plug the power cord, and close the lid into the wall. Select the CAKE course. Hit START.
6. When the add beeps, open the lid and use a rubber spatula to carefully scrape any flour left on the side of the pan. If the blade(s) are moving, please be careful.
7. Put the lid back on and keep baking. Press the START button to get the kneading going again.
8. When it's done, press CANCEL and take it out of the pan. Let it cool down before cutting it up and serving it. Enjoy!

5. MAPLE BREAD

Prep Time: 10 Minutes | Cook Time: 3 hour | Cooling Time: 2 hour

Total Times: 5 hours 10 Minutes | Serving: 4-6

Ingredients

- 2-1/4 tsp instant dry yeast.
- 1/4 cup of non-fat instant dry milk or use non-fat milk instead of water or water for dairy-free.
- 1 tbsp xanthan gum.
- 2 tbsp apple pectin.
- 1/2 cup of cornstarch.
- 1 cup of + 2 tbsp potato starch.

- 2/3 cup of brown rice flour.
- 3/4 cup of gluten-free oat flour.
- 1 tsp salt.
- 1/4 cup of pure maple syrup.
- 2 large eggs.
- 1/4 cup of more virgin olive oil that's light.
- 1-1/2 cups of + 2 tbsp water.

Instructions

1. To Make in a Bread Machine:
2. Put the wet ingredients in the bread maker's bowl and set it aside.
3. Spatula the rest of the dry ingredients together in a bowl; now, put them on top of the wet ingredients.
4. Use the instructions from the manufacturer if you have a bread machine with a gluten-free setting.
5. Help mix the ingredients first, carefully scraping the sides and bottom of the bowl. When the machine stops going up, take the paddle out of the bottom. Leave the rest to the machine. Mine takes 3 hours to do. Machines are different.
6. Also, you can top the bread with oatmeal or your favorite seeds if you want to. Use the backs of your moistened fingers to press the oatmeal and/or seeds into the dough.
7. If the kneading peddle is still in the bottom of the bread after it has been baked, take it out. Take on a wire rack and let cool for around 2 hours or until completely cool.
8. Use a knife with serrated edges, an electric meat/bread slicer with a serrated blade, or an electric knife with serrated edges to cut.
9. Make sandwiches, toast, or French toast with it. Slices that are left over can be frozen and then quickly thawed in the microwave or at room temperature.

5. CHICKPEA BREAD

Prep Time: 15-20 Minutes | Cook Time: 2-3 Minutes | Colling Time: 10 Minutes

Total Times: 2 hours 25 Minutes-3 hours 30 Minutes | Serving: 8-12

Ingredients

Wet ingredients:

- 3 large eggs, slightly beaten
- 1 1/3 cups of water
- 1 tsp cider vinegar
- 3 tbsp olive oil
- 1/4 tsp gluten-free maple flavoring extract (optional)

Dry ingredients:

- 4 tsp xanthan gum

- 3 tbsp brown sugar
- 1 cup of tapioca flour
- 1 cup of brown or white rice flour
- 1 cup of chickpea flour
- 1 (0.25 Ounce) package (7g) or 2 1/4 tsp Red Star Active Dry Yeast
- 1 1/2 tsp salt
- 1/2 cup of cornstarch
- 1/2 cup of non-fat dry milk
- 1 tbsp egg replacer (optional)

Instructions

1. Get everything to room temperature. Add the wet elements to the mixing bowl and whisk to combine. Pour the mixture into a baking pan. Place the dry elements in a separate bowl and whisk them together. Then, place the dry ingredients on top of the wet ingredients in the baking dish.
2. Choose the gluten-free cycle and turn the machine on. After the mixing starts, use a rubber spatula to work any unmixed ingredients into the dough. Keep to the edges and top of the batter to keep the kneading blade from getting in the way.
3. Take the pan out of the machine when the cycle is over. Place the bread and stay in the pan for about 10 minutes, then flip the pan over and gently shake it to get the bread out. Cool it right side up on a rack before cutting it.

7. OAT BREAD

Prep Time: 20 Minutes | Cook Time: 3 hour

Total Times: 5 hours 20 Minutes | Serving: 4-6

Ingredients

- 1/4 cup of neutral-flavored oil.
- 1 cup of + 2 tbsp of water
- 1/4 cup of non-fat instant dry milk.
- 1 tsp of gluten-free apple cider vinegar.
- 2 tbsp of honey (or sugar).
- 1 cup of + 2 tbsp potato starch.
- 1-1/2 cups of certified gluten-free oat flour.
- 3 large eggs, at room temperature(or 4 large egg whites),
- 1/2 cup of cornstarch.
- 1/4 cup of flaxseed meal.
- 1 tbsp xanthan gum.
- 1 tsp salt.
- 2-1/4 tsp instant dry yeast.
- 2 tsp gluten-free oats or seeds to sprinkle on top (optional).

Instructions

1. To make with a gluten-free setting on a bread machine:
2. Take the pan out of the bread maker. Make sure that the paddle is already on.
3. In the bowl of your bread machine, put water, dry milk, oil, vinegar, eggs, and honey.
4. Whisk the oat flour, potato starch, cornstarch, flaxseed meal, xanthan gum, yeast, and salt, if you're using them, in a separate bowl. Take all of the dry ingredients with the wet ones.
5. Put the bread pan in the machine with a snap. Choose the gluten-free option from the menu on your machine and press "Start."
6. Use a silicon spatula to remove flour from pan sides before mixing.
7. When the mixing is done, take the mixing paddle out. This will keep the bottom of your bread from getting a big hole. You use your spatula to smooth out the top.
8. If you want to put oats or seeds on top of your bread, add them now and press them in with your fingers that have been wet.
9. After the baking cycle is done, put the loaf out of the pan, then place it on a wire rack for a maximum of 2 hours to cool completely. If you don't like how crunchy the crust is, cover the top and sides with a clean tea towel while it cools on the rack. Test for desired softness. Then put it out and let it cool down all the way.
10. Once it has cooled, use a steak knife to take out the paddle. Use an electric slicer, an electric knife, or a serrated knife to cut the bread. Even though you can leave the bread out on the counter overnight, the best way to store gluten-free bread is to cut it up and freeze it.

8. POTATO BREAD WITH RICOTTA CHEESE

Prep Time: 15 Minutes | Cook Time: 2-3 hours

Total Times: 2-3 hours 15 Minutes | Serving: 8-12

Ingredients

Wet ingredients:

- 1 tsp cider vinegar
- 3/4 cup of ricotta cheese
- 1 1/4 cups of water
- 3 tbsp canola oil
- 3 large eggs, lightly beaten

Dry ingredients:

- 1/2 cup of potato starch

- 1 1/2 tsp salt
- 1/2 cup of instant potato flakes (do not pack)
- 1 tbsp xanthan gum
- 1/4 cup of granulated sugar
- 1/2 cup of tapioca flour
- 1/2 cup of cornstarch
- 1 (0.25 Ounce) package (7g) or 2 1/4 tsp
- 2 cups of brown or white rice flour
- 1/2 cup of non-fat dry milk
- 1 tbsp egg replacer (optional)

Instructions

1. Check that all of the ingredients are at room temperature. Add the wet ingredients to a bowl with a whisk, then put the mixture into a baking pan. Keep the dry ingredients in a bowl and whisk them together. Then, place the dry ingredients on top of the wet ingredients in the baking pan.
2. Choose the gluten-free cycle and turn on the machine. After the mixing starts, use a rubber spatula to work any unmixed ingredients into the dough. Stay near the edges and top of the batter to keep the kneading blade from getting in the way.
3. Take the pan out of the machine when the cycle is done. Take the bread, stay in the pan for about 10 minutes, then flip the pan over and give it a gentle shake to take the bread out. Before slicing, let it cool, standing up on a rack.

9. SOURDOUGH WHITE BREAD

Prep Time: 15 Minutes | Cook Time: 2-3 hours | Additional Time: 40 Minutes

Total Times: 2-3 hours 55 Minutes | Serving: 8-12

Ingredients

Wet ingredients:

- 3/4 cup of ricotta cheese (whole, part-skim, or non-fat)
- 1/4 cup of honey
- 3/4 cup of Gluten Free Sourdough Starter
- 1/4 cup of vegetable oil
- 1 tsp cider vinegar
- 1 cup of water
- 3 large eggs

Dry ingredients:

- 3 1/2 tsp xantham gum
- 1/2 cup of dry milk powder
- 2 cups of white rice flour
- 1 1/2 tsp salt
- 2/3 cup of potato starch
- 1/3 cup of tapioca flour

Instructions

1. Check that all of the ingredients are at room temperature. Take the wet ingredients in a bowl with a whisk, then put the mixture into a baking pan. Take the dry ingredients in a bowl and whisk them together. Then, place the dry ingredients on top of the wet ingredients in the baking pan.
2. Choose the gluten-free cycle and turn on the machine. After the mixing starts, use a rubber spatula to work any unmixed ingredients into the dough. Stay near the edges and top of the batter to keep the kneading blade from getting in the way.
3. Take the pan out of the machine when the cycle is done. Take the bread, stay in the pan for about 10 minutes, then flip the pan over and give it a gentle shake to take the bread out. Before slicing, let it cool, standing up on a rack.

10. LOW-CARB BREAD

Prep Time: 30 Minutes | Cook Time: 2-3 hours | Rising Time: 1-2 hour

Total Times: 3-5 hours 30 | Serving: 8-10

Ingredients

- 1/2 tsp bread spice
- 1 tsp salt
- 2 1/2 tsp baking powder
- 120g sunflower seeds
- 2 tbsp coconut oil
- 30g walnuts
- 230g water
- 200g ground almonds
- 10g psyllium husks

Instructions

1. First, add the dry ingredients to the bread pan. Then, add all of the liquid ingredients.
2. Choose "gluten-free cake" from the menu and press "start."
3. Then, after a few minutes, the breadmaker will beep. Push the dough down a bit, and then press the start button again.
4. After the kneading time is up, you can take out the kneading blade if you want to.
5. If you need to, use a dough scraper to shape the dough again after the kneading time.
6. Check the consistency after the program is done to see if you like it. You may bake it longer if you want to with the "Bake only" program.
7. When the bread is ready, please remove it from the pan and take it on a board.
8. Now, it cools all the way down before cutting. Enjoy!

11. MEDITERRANEAN BREAD

Prep Time: 15 Minutes | Cook Time: 2 hour

Total Times: 2 hours 15 Minutes| Serving: 8-10

Ingredients

- 250g buckwheat flour
- 200g teff flour
- 1 tbsp oil
- 1 tsp xanthan
- 2 tbsp xylitol
- 90g dried tomatoes

- 60g chopped olives
- 1 packet of dry yeast
- 100g cornstarch
- 450ml lukewarm water
- 1 tbsp psyllium husks
- 1 tsp salt

Instructions

1. In a bowl, mix the dry yeast, xylitol, and 100 ml of warm water until the yeast is dissolved. Then wait 5 to 10 minutes.
2. Make small pieces out of the dried tomatoes and olives.
3. Pour each of the dry ingredients into the Croustina bowl, and use a spatula to mix them roughly.
4. Add the yeast mixture, oil, and the rest of the lukewarm water. Use the dough scraper to mix everything together.
5. Close the Croustina and choose Program 14 for gluten-free bread. (After the time for kneading, open the lid again and, if you want, take the kneading hook out of the bowl. Now, use a dough scraper in the bowl to shape the dough again. To do this, push the dough down from the edge and toward the middle. This makes a loaf of bread with a beautiful shape. Cut three cuts in the top of the dough, and then close the Croustina lid.)
6. Let Croustina keep working in program 14 until the time for cooking and baking is up.
7. Take the bowl out of the Croustina, set the bread on a board, and bring it cool completely.
8. Let the bread cool a little bit before slicing it. Enjoy!

12. PALEO BREAD

Prep Time: 15 Minutes | Cook Time: 3 hours

Total Times: 3 hours 15 Minutes | Serving: 8-12

Ingredients

- 4 Tbsp Chia seeds
- 2 tsp cream of tartar
- 1 ¼ Cups of tapioca flour
- 1 tsp Real Salt
- ¾ Cup of + 1 Tbsp water
- 2 tsp bread machine yeast
- ½ Cup of almond milk
- 2 Cups of almond flour

- 1 tsp baking soda
- 1 Tbsp flax meal
- 3 eggs (room temperature)
- 1 Tbsp maple syrup or honey
- ¼ Cups of flax meal
- ⅓ Cup of coconut flour
- ¼ Cup of coconut oil

Instructions

1. In a bowl, mix it with the Chia seeds and the tbsp of flax meal. Mix the water in and set it aside. As the mixture sits, it will turn into a gel.
2. Melt the coconut oil and allow it cool until it is about room temperature. Mix in the eggs, almond milk, and honey or maple syrup.
3. Mix in the gel made from Chia seeds and flax meal. When everything is mixed well, pour it into the bread maker's pan.
4. Mix the almond flour, tapioca flour, coconut flour, salt, and 1/4 cup of flax meal together.
5. Cream of tartar and baking soda need to be mixed together well. Combine it well with the other dry ingredients.
6. Fill the bread machine with the dry ingredients. On top, make a small well and add the yeast.
7. For a 2-pound loaf, turn the machine on to the Whole Grain setting.

13. CINNAMON, FRUIT, AND RAISIN BREAD

Prep Time: 15 Minutes | Cook Time: 2 hours

Total Times: 2 hours 15 Minutes | Serving: 14

Ingredients

- 2/3 cup of potato starch
- 1/3 cup of tapioca starch
- 1 tbsp xanthan gum
- 1 tsp plain gelatin
- 1 tbsp ground cinnamon
- 2 tsp bread machine yeast
- 3/4 cup of raisins
- 1 tsp salt
- 3 tbsp brown sugar

- 2 tbsp skim milk powder
- 2 cups of rice flour
- 1 1/3 cups of water
- 3 large eggs
- 3 tbsp melted margarine or 3 tbsp butter
- 2/3 cup of mashed ripe bananas or 2/3 cup of applesauce

Instructions

1. Add the first four ingredients to the pan of the bread machine and mix well with a plastic whisk or fork. Take the rest of the ingredients in the order shown. Choose either the rapid or basic white cycle (which takes about 2 to 3 hours.)
2. After 5 minutes of mixing, use a rubber spatula or silicone spatula to scrape down the sides of the pan. When the bread is done, put it out of the pan and take it on a rack.
3. TIP: Use 1/4 cup of chopped nuts instead of 1/4 cup of raisins.
4. Add 1 tsp of white vinegar or cider vinegar if you use instant yeast.
5. Use a super-express cycle (1 to 1 1/4 hours) to try this recipe.
6. Potato flour should not be used instead of potato starch.
7. Making bread in a machine is easy.

14. WHITE BREAD

Prep Time: 15 Minutes | Rising time: 1 hour | Cook Time: 2 hours

Total Times: 3 hours 15 Minutes | Serving: 8-12

Ingredients

Medium Loaf :

- 2 tbsp Sugar
- 2 tsp quick yeast
- 1 tsp Salt
- 450g FREEE White Bread Flour
  2 cups

- 1 tsp vinegar
- 6 tbsp oil
- 310ml milk *1 1/3 cups*
- 2 eggs

Instructions

1. Take the eggs in a large bowl and beat them well.
2. Mix the milk, oil, and vinegar together well with a whisk.
3. Put this into the pan for the bread machine.
4. Add the salt, sugar, and flour.
5. The yeast goes on top.
6. Make sure the pan is locked in place, and put the lid on.
7. If there is a gluten-free bread setting, use that. If not, use the basic rapid set.
8. Choose the dark crust if it's an option.
9. Get the machine going.
10. When the bread is done baking, carefully take the pan out of the machine.
11. Put the bread out of the pan and take the mixer paddle out of the bottom of the loaf.
12. On a wire rack, let the bread cool.
13. Wait until the bread is cold before cutting it for the best results.

15. BROWN BREAD

Prep Time: 15 Minutes | Rising time: 1 hour | Cook Time: 2 hour

Total Times: 3 hours 15 Minutes | Serving: 8-12

Ingredients

Medium Loaf :

- 2 tbsp Sugar
- 2 tsp quick yeast
- 1 tsp Salt
- 500g FREEE Brown Bread Flour
- 1 tsp vinegar
- 6 tbsp oil
- 530ml milk
- 2 eggs

Instructions

1. Whisk the egg whites, milk, oil, and vinegar together in a bowl.
2. Put this into the pan for the bread machine.
3. Add the sugar, salt, and flour.
4. The yeast goes on top.
5. Make sure the pan is locked in place, and put the lid on.
6. If you can, use the gluten-free bread program. If not, use a basic rapid setting.
7. Choose the dark crust if it's an option.
8. Get the machine going.
9. When the bread is done baking, carefully take the pan out of the machine.
10. Put the bread out of the pan and take the paddle from the bottom of the loaf.
11. On a wire rack, let the bread cool.
12. Wait until the bread is cold before cutting it for the best results.

16. MULTIGRAIN BREAD

Prep Time: 15 Minutes | Cook Time: 3 hours

Total Times: 3 hours 15 Minutes | Serving: 8-10

Ingredients

- 1-1/4 cups of + 1 tbsp water, heated to 80 - 110°F.
- 1 tsp salt.
- 1-3/4 tsp instant dry yeast.
- 2 tbsp psyllium husk powder.
- 2 tbsp golden flaxseed meal.
- 2 tbsp gluten-free protein powder such as brown rice protein.
- 2 tbsp millet flour.
- 1/4 cup of buckwheat flour.
- 1 cup of brown rice flour.
- 1-1/4 cups of cornstarch.
- 1 tsp apple cider vinegar.
- 2 large egg whites.
- 3 tbsp of Lyle's Golden Syrup (or light corn syrup).
- 1/3 cup of sunflower oil.
- 1/4 cup of + 2 tbsp (6 tbsp) unsweetened applesauce.
- 2 tsp sunflower seeds, plus more seeds of choice for the top (optional).
- 1/2 tsp guar gum (optional if you are intolerant).

Instructions

1. Pour all the liquid ingredients into the bread machine's bowl.
2. The remaining dry ingredients can be mixed together in a separate bowl.
3. Put the dry mixture on top of the wet mixture and follow the directions on your bread machine.
4. Move the bread right away to a wire rack to cool completely, which will take about 2 hours.
5. Use an electric slicer, a knife with serrated edges, or an electric knife to cut.

17. SORGHUM BREAD

Prep Time: 20 Minutes | Cook Time: 1 hour 20 Minutes

Total Times: 3 hours 40 Minutes | Serving: 8-10

Ingredients

- 1 cup of + 2 tbsp water at room temperature.
- 1 tsp salt.
- 2-1/4 tsp instant dry yeast.
- 1 tbsp xanthan gum.
- 1/2 cup of cornstarch (or tapioca flour).
- 1 cup of + 2 tbsp potato starch.
- 1-1/2 cups of certified gluten-free oat flour, plus more for dusting.
- 2 tbsp honey (or sugar).
- 2 large egg whites.
- 2 large eggs.
- 1 tsp gluten-free apple cider vinegar.
- 1/4 cup of neutral-flavored oil.
- 1/4 cup of non-fat instant dry mil

Instructions

1. To make with a gluten-free setting on a bread machine:
2. Get the pan out of the bread machine. Make sure that the paddle is already in place.
3. Pour water, dry milk, oil, vinegar, eggs, and honey into the bread machine's bowl.
4. Whisk the oat flour, potato starch, cornstarch, xanthan gum, yeast, and salt, if using, in a separate bowl. Add up the dry ingredients to the wet ones.
5. Put the bread pan into the machine with a snap. Choose the gluten-free option from your machine's menu and press "Start."
6. At the start of the mixing cycle, use a silicone spatula to scrape the flour off the pan's sides.
7. Take out the mixing paddle when the mixing cycle is done. This will keep your bread from getting a big hole in the bottom. Use your spatula to smooth the top.
8. If you want to put oats or seeds on top of your bread, add them now and press them into the dough with wet fingers.
9. When the baking cycle is done, Put the loaf out of the pan and take it on a wire rack for a maximum of 2 hours to cool completely. If you don't like how crunchy the crust is, cover the top and sides with a clean tea towel while it cools on the rack. Test for desired softness. Then put it out and let it cool down completely.
10. Once it has cooled, use a steak knife to take out the paddle (if you left it in). Use an electric slicer, a knife, or an electric knife with serrated edges to cut the bread. Even though you can leave the bread out on the counter overnight, you should always slice and freeze gluten-free bread.

18. BARLEY BREAD

Prep Time: 10 Minutes | Cook Time: 1-2 hours

Total Times: 1-2 hour 10 minutes

Serving: 8-10

Ingredients

- 1 tsp xanthan gum
- 1 cup of rice flour
- 3/4 cup of warm water (100-115 degrees F)
- 1 tsp salt
- 5 tsp yeast
- 3 Tbsp sugar
- 4 Tbsp rice milk
- 1 cup of barley flour
- 1/4 cup of tapioca starch
- 1 Tbsp oil

Instructions

1. Combine rice flour, barley flour, tapioca starch, and xanthan gum. Follow the bread machine's instructions to add the ingredients. Bake on a "super rapid" cycle or equivalent. Makes 1 pound loaf.

19. HIGH PROTEIN GLUTEN FREE BREAD

Prep Time: 20 Minutes | Cook Time: 3 hours

Total Times: 5 hours 20 Minutes | Serving: 12

Ingredients

- 1 cup of + 2 tbsp water at room temperature.
- 1 tsp salt.
- 2-1/4 tsp instant dry yeast.
- 1 tbsp xanthan gum.
- 1/4 cup of shelled hemp seeds.
- 1/4 cup of flaxseed meal.
- 1/2 cup of cornstarch.
- 1 cup of + 2 tbsp potato starch.
- 1-1/2 cups of certified gluten-free oat flour
- 2 tbsp full-flavored molasses(honey)
- 3 large eggs at room temperature. (or 4 large egg whites),
- 1 tsp gluten-free apple cider vinegar.
- 1/4 cup of neutral-flavored oil.
- 1/3 cup of non-fat instant dry milk.
- 2 tsp gluten-free oats or seeds for topping (optional).

Instructions

1. To make with a gluten-free setting on a bread machine.Take the pan out of the bread maker.Make sure that the paddle is already on.In the bowl of your bread machine, put water, dry milk, oil, vinegar, eggs, and molasses.
2. Whisk the oat flour, potato starch, cornstarch, xanthan gum, yeast, and salt, if you're using them, in a separate bowl. Put the dry ingredients with the wet ones.
3. Put the bread pan in the machine with a snap. Choose the gluten-free option from the menu on your machine and press "Start."
4. At the outset of the mixing process, use a silicone spatula to remove the flour from the pan's sides.
5. When the mixing is done, take the mixing paddle out. This will keep the bottom of your bread from getting a big hole. You use your spatula to smooth out the top.
6. If you want to put oats or seeds on top of your bread, add them now and press them in with your fingers that have been wet.
7. After the baking cycle is done, Put the loaf out of the pan and take it on a wire rack for a maximum of 2 hours to cool completely. Use a fresh tea towel to cover the top and sides of the crust while it cools on the rack if the crust is too crunchy for you. Test for desired softness. Then put it out and let it cool down all the way.
8. Remove the paddle with a steak knife after cooling. Cut bread with a serrated knife, electric knife, or slicer. Gluten-free bread should be cut up and frozen rather than left on the counter overnight.

20. OAT & RICE BREAD

Prep Time: 10 Minutes | Cook Time: 1 hour 30 Minutes

Total Times: 3 hours 45 Minutes | Serving: 8-12

Ingredients

- 1 cup of + 2 tbsp water.
- 2-1/4 tsp instant dry yeast.
- 1/4 cup of non-fat instant dry milk.
- 1 tbsp xanthan gum.
- 1/4 cup of flaxseed meal
- 1/2 cup of cornstarch
- 1 cup of + 2 tbsp potato starch.
- 1/2 cup of brown rice flour
- 3/4 cup of gluten-free oat flour
- 1 tsp sea salt
- 1 tsp gluten-free apple cider vinegar
- 2 tbsp honey (or sugar).
- 3 large eggs at room temperature.
- 1/4 cup of light virgin olive oil (or oil of choice)
- 2 tsp gluten-free oats on top (optional)

Instructions

1. Put the wet ingredients in the bread maker's bowl and set it aside.
2. Add the remaining dry ingredients on top of the wet ones after combining them in a separate bowl.
3. Take the directions from the manufacturer if you have a bread machine with a gluten-free setting.
4. If you have a programmable bread machine that doesn't have a gluten-free setting, set it to Crust: Medium; Keep Warm: 0; 1st Knead: 5 minutes; 2nd Knead: 10 minutes; 1st Rise: 40 minutes; Punch: 10 minutes; 2nd Rise: 10 minutes; Shape: 5 minutes; 3rd Rise: 35 minutes; Bake: 65 to 90 minutes. The same goes for one or

two rises. Just make sure that the final rise is long and that the bread is nice and high.

5. After stirring my machine for 15 to 20 minutes, I open it and use a silicone spatula to remove any loose flour from the sides and bottom. For machines that don't make gluten-free food, you can do this however you want. Let the rest be done by the machine. Total time: 2 hours, 50 minutes to 3 hours, depending on the machine.

6. If you don't want a big hole at the bottom, you can take the paddle out of the machine after the stirring is done. Also, you can top the bread with oatmeal or your favorite seeds if you want to. Use the backs of your moistened fingers to press the oatmeal and/or seeds into the dough.

7. If the kneading peddle is still in the bottom of the bread after it has been baked, take it out. Put on a wire rack and let it cool for around 2 hours or until completely cool.

8. Use a knife with serrated edges, an electric meat/bread slicer with a serrated blade, or an electric knife with serrated edges to cut.

9. Make sandwiches, toast, or French toast with it. Slices that are left over can be frozen and then quickly thawed in the microwave or at room temperature.

21. SOURDOUGH BREAD

Prep Time: 20 Minutes | Cook Time: 1 hour 30 Minutes

Total Times: 3 hours 50 Minutes | Serving: 8-10

Ingredients

- 2 tbsp water
- 2-1/4 cups of Carla's Gluten Free Sourdough Starter
- 1/2 cup of brown rice flour
- 1/16 tsp citric acid (recommended but may be omitted)
- 1-1/4 tsp salt.
- 2 tsp instant dry yeast
- 1 tbsp xanthan gum.
- 1/2 cup of cornstarch
- 1 cup of + 2 tbsp potato starch
- 2-1/2 tbsp granulated sugar, organic if desired (or honey)
- 2 large egg whites
- 1/4 cup of neutral-flavored oil

Instructions

1. Mix the sourdough starter, water, and brown rice flour together with a whisk. Set the mixture aside to ferment for 1–4 hours or until it starts to bubble.
2. To make with a gluten-free setting on a bread machine
3. Add the oil, rice flour, sourdough starter, eggs, sugar, or honey, and set aside.
4. Potato starch, cornstarch, xanthan gum, yeast, and salt should be whisked together in a medium-sized bowl. Add the citric acid if you want a sour taste. Using 1/32 will only make the taste a little bit sour. So, for more, use 1/16.
5. Put the dry ingredients into the bread maker. Set the machine to "Gluten Free," bake as directed, and press the "Start" button. Help stir the mixture with a silicone spatula so that all of the dry flour gets wet. After mixing is done, and the dough starts to rise, you can take the mixing paddle out if you want to.
6. To mix, let rise, and bake; it takes 3 hours.
7. Take the bread out of the machine right away. Move it to a wire rack and put it cool for 2 hours.

22. YEAST-BASED PALEO BREAD

Prep Time: 5 Minutes | Cook Time: 2-3 Minutes | Rising time: 1-2 hour

Total Times: 3 hours 5 Minutes-5 hours 5 Minutes Serving: 8-12

Ingredients

- ¼ cup of Extra Virgin Coconut Oil
- 7/8 cups of Mineral Water
- 2/3 cup of Tapioca Flour
- 2 Tbsp Honey
- ½ cup of Golden Flaxseed Meal(it's the same as 220mL or you can measure 1 cup of and remove 2 Tbsp)
- 2/3 cup of Arrowroot Flour
- 1 tsp Salt
- 4 cups of Blanched Almond Flour
- 2 eggs
- 2 tsp Active Dry Yeast
- 1 Tbsp Apple Cider Vinegar

Instructions

1. Fill the bottom of your Bread Machine pan, mix mineral water, eggs, ground flaxseed, salt, honey, and vinegar. Take a fork, break up the eggs, and mix the ground flaxseed well. Let sit for 2 minutes before adding the dry ingredients.
2. On top of the wet elements, add the coconut oil, almond flour, tapioca flour, and arrowroot flour. Sprinkle yeast on top of the flour, or follow the instructions for your bread machine.
3. Set your Bread Machine to the whole wheat setting. During the first kneading, make sure that the ingredients are mixing well and that none of them are sticking to the edge of the pan.
4. Take the bread out of the machine as soon as it's done. Enjoy!

23. WHOLEMEAL BREAD

Prep Time: 10 Minutes | Cook Time: 1 hour 50 Minutes

Total Times: 2 hours | Serving: 12

Ingredients

Dry Ingredients:

- 20 g additional tapioca starch flour
- 200 g Gluten Free Alchemist Rice Free Flour Blend
- 5 g INSTANT Easy Bake fast action yeast
- 24 g milk powder/coconut milk powder omit if using liquid milk in place of water (below)
- 8 g fine sea salt
- 18 g milled flax seed
- 35 g ground psyllium husk grind in a blender (not 'psyllium powder')
- 140 g gluten-free oat flour

Wet Ingredients:

- 3 large eggs UK large, maximum liquid weight 168g (minimum 163g) better to aim towards lower weight end of 163g in most machines
- 1 tbsp(24) g honey or maple syrup
- 325 g hand-warm water or milk (dairy or DF)
- 2 tbsp (30g)sunflower or olive oil
- 1 tsp (5)g lemon juice

Instructions

Dry Ingredients:

1. Weigh and mix all the dry ingredients together, then set them aside. TIP: Put the weight in a container that can't let air in and shake it hard.
2. Put the yeast pot or sachet next to the other dry ingredients so it doesn't get left out.

Wet Ingredients:

1. Take all the wet ingredients in a bowl and put a hand whisk to mix them all together.
2. Bake in the Breadmaker:
3. Make sure the paddle is in the bread machine before you start.
4. Take the liquid ingredients to the bread machine.
5. Mix together the yeast and the dry ingredients quickly.
6. Take the dry ingredients on top of the wet ingredients in the bowl of the bread machine.
7. Set the bread machine to GF and press the "start" button.
8. While your bread is baking, have a cup of tea and read a magazine while enjoying the smell of a freshly baked yeast loaf.
9. Once the bread is done, put it out of the bread machine and carefully slide it out sideways so you don't squash the top. Put on a wire rack to cool.
10. Once the paddle is cool, carefully take it out.

24. CINNAMON RAISIN BREAD

Prep Time: 10 Minutes | Cook Time: 2 hours

Total Times: 2 hours 10 Minutes | Serving: 8

Ingredients

- 3 tbsp granulated sugar
- 3 large eggs, room temperature
- 2 tsp active yeast
- 1 tbsp of xanthan gum (if you do not have xanthan gum, you can substitute 3 tbsp of psyllium husk powder instead.)
- 4 tbsp of (1/2 stick) unsalted butter, room temperature
- 3 1/4 cups of gluten-free, all-purpose flour (442 g if using Bob's Red Mill Flour)
- 1 cup of water, warm

For the cinnamon sugar mixture:

- 2 tsp ground cinnamon
- 1/4 cup of granulated sugar
- 1/4 cup of raisins (if you are not a fan of raisins, feel free to leave them out)

Instructions

1. Prepare the yeast by putting the yeast, warm water, and sugar in a bowl and stirring them together. Put the mixture aside until it gets foamy—about 5 minutes.
2. Check that all of the ingredients are at room temperature, then put the butter, eggs, and yeast mixture in the bread machine's baking pan.
3. Pour in the gluten-free flour, then the xanthan gum, and then the salt.
4. Set the bread machine to the setting for gluten-free bread and press the "start" button.
5. When the paddle signal sounds, press the start/stop button, open the lid, and Onto a piece of parchment paper or plastic wrap that has been dusted with flour, pour the dough. Make a square with the dough.
6. In a bowl, mix with the sugar, cinnamon, and raisins. Then, sprinkle the mixture over the bread dough.
7. Lift up one side of the plastic wrap and gently pull the dough up so it forms a log.
8. Using both sides of the plastic wrap, put the dough log right into the baking pan of the bread machine.Press the start button again, and then let the machine do its thing.
9. When the bread is done, slide it out of the bread pan and onto a wire rack. Let it cool before you cut it. Enjoy!

25. APPLE SPICE BREAD

Prep Time: 10-15 Minutes | Cook Time: 2-3 hours

Total Times: 2-3 hours 10-15 Minutes | Serving: 8-12

Ingredients

- ½ Cup of(s) Pecan Pieces
- 1 Active Dry Yeast Packet
- ¾ Cup of(s)Brown Rice Flour
- ¾ Cup of(s)Tapioca Flour
- ¾ Cup of(s Millet Flour
- ½ Cup of(s) Corn Starch
- 2 Tbsp Apple Pie Spice
- 1 Tbsp Xanthan Gum
- 1 Tsp Salt
- 3 Eggs, room temperature, slightly beaten
- 1 Cup of(s) Granny Smith Apples, grated
- ½ Cup of(s) Warm Water (85-95°F)
- 3 Tbsp Light Brown Suger, packed
- 3 Tbsp Canola Oil
- 1 Tsp Cider Vinegar

Instructions

1. Mix brown rice and tapioca flour, milk powder, potato starch, soy flour, sugar, cinnamon, xanthan gum, and salt in a bowl. Set aside.
2. Eggs, apples, water, brown sugar, oil, and vinegar are mixed together, then poured into a bread pan. Pour the flour mixture over the liquids and sprinkle yeast on top.
3. Put the bread pan in the baking chamber, close the lid, and plug the bread maker into the wall. Choose BASIC SETTING, 2POUND LOAF, MEDIUM CRUST. Then press the START button.
4. When the "add ingredient" beep sounds, put the nuts right into the bread pan. After the bread has finished baking, put it out of the pan and take it on a wire rack.
5. Cool, all the way. To serve, cut into slices.

26. CHERRY BREAD

Prep Time: 15 Minutes | Cook Time: 15-30 Minutes

Total Times: 30-45 Minutes | Serving: 8-10

Ingredients

- 2 Tbsp organic cherry juice
- 1/2 cup of dried cherries
- 1 cup of natural applesauce
- 1 tsp sea salt
- 6 Ounce soy milk
- 2 1/2 cups of flour (or sweet bread flour)
- 3/4 cup of sugar
- 3 1/2 tsp safe baking powder

Instructions

1. Bring milk to room temperature or heat it in the microwave for 15–20 seconds. Add to bread pan. Applesauce and cherry juice can be added. Take the flour, sugar, baking powder, and salt in a medium bowl. Mix well, then put in the bread pan. Toss in cherries. Use the setting for quick bread. Turn the machine to bake only when it's done. Check on your bread every five minutes until the middle is no longer doughy. In my bread machine, this takes about 15 minutes longer.

27. HAWAIIAN SWEET BREAD

Prep Time: 5 Minutes | Cook Time: 2 hours 6 Minutes

Total Times: 2 hours 33 Minutes | Serving: 8-12

Ingredients

- 3/4 cup of pineapple juice
- 3/4 tsp salt
- 3 eggs beaten
- 2 1/2 tsp sugar
- 2 tbsp milk
- 1 1/2 tsp Fleischmann's Bread Machine Instant Yeast
- 2 tbsp olive oil
- 3 cups of Bob Mills 1:1 Gluten Free Flour

Instructions

2. My bread machine says to put all the wet ingredients in first, so I did that. Before putting in the flour, I mix the yeast and flour together to make sure it goes in evenly.
3. I put my bread basket back in the cup of board and lock it.
4. Then, I choose the gluten-free setting and set the crust color to middle or dark.
5. After the second rise, I check to see if all the flour and the dough look like they are mixed well.
6. I then let the machine do its job and wait longingly for it to complete.
7. I take the basket out and let it cool for around 20 minutes on a wire rack.

28. AUTUMN PUMPKIN BREAD

Prep Time: 15 Minutes | Cook Time: 2-3 hours

Total Times: 2-3 hours 15 Minutes | Serving: 8-12

Ingredients

- 1 ml (1/4 tsp) ground allspice
- 45 ml (3 tbsp) light olive oil
- 5 ml (1 tsp) ground cinnamon
- 75 g (1/3 cup of) cane sugar
- 1 ml (1/4 tsp) ground nutmeg
- 60 ml (4 tbsp) plant-based milk
- ml (1 1/2 tsp) instant yeast
- 70 g (1/2 cup of) pumpkin seeds
- 385 g (or 2 3/4 cups of) all-purpose flour "La Merveilleuse"
- 375 g (1 1/2 cups of) pumpkin puree
- 2 large eggs (110 g))
- 30 ml (2 tbsp) maple syrup
- 3.5ml (3/4 tsp) salt
- 80 g (1/2 cup of) semi-sweet chocolate chips
- 20 g (30 ml / 2 tbsp) chia seeds

Instructions

1. Use a coffee grinder to make the chia powder.
2. Mix the ground chia, flour, sugar, spices, salt, and baking powder together in a bowl. Set aside.
3. Heat the pumpkin puree and plant-based milk substitute in a small saucepan until they reach the right temperature for your bread maker.
4. Place the pan off the heat and add the eggs, oil, and maple syrup. Then whisk the mixture very hard. Check that the kneading blade is in the bread machine correctly, and then pour the liquid ingredients into the machine.
5. Add the dry ingredients, and then, depending on the brand and model of your own bread machine, start the machine on the right cycle.
6. Wait about 2 minutes, then open the lid and take a spatula to scrape the sides so that all of the flour gets mixed in.
7. Close the lid then the machine runs until it sounds an alert to add ingredients. When this signal goes off, open the lid, add the chocolate chips and pumpkin seeds, close the lid, and let the machine finish its full cycle. Note: Each bread machine has a different sound that tells you when to add ingredients. Check your manual for the exact time.
8. When the cycle is done, take the bread out, take it out of the pan, then it cools completely on a wire rack. Don't take the kneading blade out of the bread until it has completely cooled down.

29. ZUCCHINNI BREAD

Prep Time: 15 Minutes | Cook Time: 1-2 hours

Total Times: 1-2 hours | Serving: 8-12

Ingredients

- 1/3 cup of oil
- 1/3 cup of packed brown sugar
- 3 T. granulated sugar
- 2 eggs
- 1/2 tsp baking soda
- 3/4 tsp salt
- 1/2 tsp baking powder
- 3/4 tsp. cinnamon
- 1 1/2 cup of gluten-free Featherlite flour
- 3/4 cup of zucchini, shredded
- 1/4 tsp allspice
- 1/3 cup of walnuts (optional)
- 1/3 cup of raisins (optional)

Instructions

1. Add all of the ingredients into a bread machine pan that has been sprayed with Pam. For quick bread, press the menu button. Enjoy!

30. BANANA AND HEMP BREAD

Prep Time: 15 Minutes | Cook Time: 1-2 hours

Total Times: 1-2 hour 15 Minutes | Serving: 8-10

Ingredients

- 2 tbsp (30m/20 g) chia seeds
- 3/4 tsp(3,5 ml) salt
- 4 tbsp(60 ml) plant-based milk
- 2 tbsp (30 ml) maple syrup
- 1/3 cup of(40g) hemp seeds
- 1/4 tsp (1ml) ground nutmeg
- 1 1/2 cup of (420g) crushed ripe bananas

- 1/2 cup of (80g) semi-sweet chocolate chips
- 3 tbsp (45ml) light olive oil
- 2 3/4 cups of (385g) all-purpose flour
- 1/4 tsp (1ml) instant yeast
- 2 large eggs (110 g)
- (1/2 cup of (110g) cane sugar

Instructions

2. Use a coffee grinder to make the chia powder.
3. Mix the dry ingredients: ground chia, flour, sugar, nutmeg, salt, and instant yeast in a large bowl. Set aside.
4. Mix the mashed bananas, plant-based milk substitute, oil, and maple syrup in a small saucepan.
5. Heat to the temperature that your bread machine model calls for.
6. Put the pan off the heat, add the eggs, and whisk the mixture very well. Check that the kneading blade is in the bread machine correctly, then pour the liquid ingredients into the machine.
7. Place the dry ingredients you saved on top, and then, depending on the brand and model of your bread machine, start the machine on the right cycle.
8. Wait about 2 minutes, then open the lid and take a spatula to scrape the sides so that all of the flour gets mixed in.
9. Close the lid and let the machine keep going until it beeps to tell you to add ingredients. When you hear the signal, open the lid and take the chocolate chips and hemp seeds. Close the lid, then let the machine finish its full cycle.
10. When the cycle is over, take the bread out, take it out of the pan, and it cools completely on a wire rack. Don't take the kneading blade out of the bread until it has completely cooled down.

31. BREAD RECIPE WITHOUT FLAXSEED MEAL

Prep Time: 15 Minutes | Cook Time: 1 hour 30 Minutes

Total Times: 3 hours 45 Minutes | Serving: 10-12

Ingredients

- 1 tsp apple cider vinegar
- 1-1/2 cups of + 2 tbsp water
- 2-1/4 tsp instant dry yeast
- 3/4 cup of gluten-free oat flour (or 2/3 cup of sorghum flour)
- 1/4 cup of non-fat instant dry milk (or use non-fat milk instead of water or water for dairy-free)
- 2/3 cup of brown rice flour
- 3 large eggs (or 1/2 cup of) at room temperature
- 2 tbsp of honey (or agave or sugar)
- 2 tbsp apple pectin 1 tbsp xanthan gum (or guar gum for corn-free)
- 1 cup of + 2 tbsp of potato starch 1/2 cup of cornstarch (or tapioca flour/starch)
- 1/4 cup of light virgin olive oil (or oil of choice)
- 1 tsp salt

Instructions

1. Put the wet ingredients in the bread maker's bowl and set it aside.
2. Take the remaining dry ingredients to the wet ones after combining them in a separate bowl.
3. Follow the manufacturer's directions when using a bread machine with a gluten-free setting. If you have a programmable bread machine that doesn't have a gluten-free setting, set it to Crust: Medium; Keep Warm: 0; 1st Knead: 5 minutes; 2nd Knead: 10 minutes; 1st Rise: 40 minutes; Punch: 10 minutes; 2nd Rise: 10 minutes; Shape: 5 minutes; 3rd Rise: 35 minutes; Bake: 65 to 90 minutes. The same goes for one or two rises. Just make sure that the final rise is long and that the bread is nice and high.
4. After stirring my machine for 15 to 20 minutes, I open it and use a silicone spatula to remove any loose flour from the sides and bottom. For machines that don't make gluten-free food, you can do this however you want. Let the rest be done by the machine. Total time: 2 hours, 50 minutes to 3 hours, depending on the machine.
5. If you don't want a big hole in the bottom of your bread, you can take the paddle out of the machine after the stirring is done. Also, you can top the bread with oatmeal or your favorite seeds if you want to. Use the backs of your moistened fingers to press the oatmeal and/or seeds into the dough.
6. If the kneading peddle is still in the bottom of the bread after it has been baked, take it out. Take on a wire rack and let cool for around 2 hours or until completely cool.

7. Use a knife with serrated edges, an electric meat/bread slicer with a serrated blade, or an electric knife with serrated edges to cut.
8. Make sandwiches, toast, or French toast with it. Slices that are left over can be frozen and then quickly thawed in the microwave or at room temperature.

32. GREEN TEA BREAD

Prep Time: 15 Minutes | Cook Time: 2-4 Minutes

Total Times: 2-4 hours 15 Minutes | Serving: 8-12

Ingredients

- 3 large eggs, beaten
- 1-1/2 cups of (360mL) milk
- 1-1/2 cups of (210g) potato starch
- 1 tsp. (5.6g) salt
- 1/8 cup of (27g) vegetable oil
- 1 Tbsp. (8g) xanthan gum
- 2-1/2 cups of (370g) brown rice flour
- 2 Tbsp. (40g) honey
- 1 Tbsp. (8.5g) active dry yeast
- 1 tsp. (3g) matcha (powdered green tea)
- 1 Tbsp. (14mL) apple cider vinegar

Instructions

1. With a whisk, mix the potato starch, brown rice flour, xanthan gum, and green tea powder together well in a large bowl.
2. Make sure the kneading blades are properly attached, and then add the milk, beaten eggs, apple cider vinegar, vegetable oil, and honey.
3. Add the mixture of flour and salt from the previous step l to the baking pan. Take a spoon, make a small hole in the flour, and put the yeast there. Make sure the yeast doesn't get in contact with the liquid and salt.
4. Put the pan into the Home Bakery.
5. Set the control for the crust, and then press START. When the add beeps, use a rubber spatula to push any flour stuck to the sides down. If the blades that knead the dough are moving, please be careful.
6. Press and hold the START/RESET or CANCEL button to turn the unit off when baking is done. Put the bread right away on a rack to cool.
7. Let the bread cool down. Cut it up and serve.

33. BRIOCHE BREAD

Prep Time: 15 Minutes | Cook Time: 2-3 hours

Total Times: 2-3 hours 15 minutes | Serving: 8-12

Ingredients

- 2 1/2 cups of + 2 tbsp gluten-free all-purpose flour
- 1 packet of granulated yeast
- 1 cup of whole milk
- 2 tsp xanthan gum
- 2 tsp sea salt
- 4 tbsp salted butter
- 1/4 cups of sugar
- 2 extra-large eggs

Instructions

1. Take the milk, butter, sugar, and salt in a measuring cup of with 2 cups of. Heat in the microwave for around 1 1/2 minutes or until the milk is steaming and the butter has melted. Pour the mixture into the bread machine's pan. Using a fork, vigorously whisk the eggs in the same two-cup of measure, then add them to the bread pan. Put the flour on top of the wet ingredients in the pan and sprinkle the xanthan gum on top of the flour. Do not stir. Get a shallow well in the middle of the flour with your index finger and put the granulated yeast in the well.

2. Put the bread pan into the bread machine and make sure it's in place the way the manufacturer tells you to. Close the lid and press the "menu" or "select" button. You should choose the "basic/white bread" cycle. Choose "1 1/2-pound loaf" by pressing the "loaf size" button. Click on "light crust" on the "crust control" button. Press the "start" button. Depending on the length of the loaf you are making and the make and model of your bread machine, the whole baking process will take about 2 1/2-3 hours. Walk away. Do not lift the lid to see how things are going. When the machine beeps to let you know it's done, carefully open the lid. Using pot holders or oven mitts, take the bread pan out of the machine by lifting it by its handle. Turn the bread pan at about a 30-45 degree angle and gently shake or slide the loaf out onto its side. Turn the loaf over and put it on a cooling rack so it can cool all the way down. If the kneading paddle is still in the loaf after it is taken out of the pan, I find it easiest to take it out after the loaf has cooled for 5–10 minutes.

34. BUTTER PECAN SUPREME BREAD

Prep Time: 15 Minutes Cook Time: 1-2 hours

Total Times: 1-2 hour 15 minutes | Serving: 8-12

Ingredients

Wet ingredients:

- 1 tsp cider vinegar
- 2 tbsp butter (room temperature)
- 1 cup of plus 1 tbsp of water (room temperature)
- 3 large eggs, lightly beaten (room temperature)

Dry ingredients:

- 1 1/2 tbsp xanthan gum
- 1 1/2 tsp salt
- 1/2 cup of tapioca flour
- 1 (0.25 Ounce) package (7g) or 2 1/4 tsp Red Star Active Dry Yeast
- 3/4 cup of pecan meal
- 1/4 cup of brown sugar
- 1/2 cup of potato starch
- 1 1/2 cups of rice flour
- 1 tbsp egg replacer (optional)

Instructions

1. Check to make sure that everything is at room temperature. Add the wet ingredients to a bowl with a whisk, then put the mixture into a baking pan. Take the dry ingredients in a separate bowl and whisk them together. Then, take the dry ingredients on top of the wet ingredients in the baking pan.
2. Choose the gluten-free cycle and turn on the machine. After the mixing starts, use a rubber spatula to work any unmixed ingredients into the dough. Stay near the edges and top of the batter to keep the kneading blade from getting in the way.
3. Take the pan out of the machine when the cycle is done. Take the bread, stay in the pan for about 10 minutes, then flip the pan over and give it a gentle shake to take the bread out. Before slicing, let it cool, standing up on a rack.

35. SUN DRIED TOMATO BREAD

Prep Time: 10 Minutes | Cook Time: 1 Hour 30 Minutes

Total Times: 1 Hour 40 Minutes | Serving: 12 Slice

Ingredients

- 1/2 cup of cornstarch or tapioca flour/starch
- 3/4 cup of gluten-free oat flour or 2/3 cup of sorghum flour
- 3 large eggs
- 1 tbsp sea salt
- 1 cup of + 2 tbsp potato
- 1/2 cup of at room temperature
- 1/4 cup of drained sun-dried tomatoes in oil & Italian herbs (45g)
- 1 tsp gluten-free apple cider vinegar
- 2 tbsp honey or agave or sugar
- 1/2 cup of + 2 tbsp of brown rice flour
- 1/4 cup of flaxseed meal golden and/or brown
- 1/4 cup of light virgin olive oil or oil of choice
- 1 cup of + 2 tbsp water

Instructions

1. Put the wet ingredients in the bread maker bowl and set it aside.
2. Place the wet ingredients in the bread maker bowl and set it aside.
3. Follow the manufacturer directions when using a bread machine with a gluten-free setting. For gluten-free bread, I use setting number 10 on my Breadman BK1050S.
4. After stirring my machine for 15 to 20 minutes, I open it and use a silicone spatula to remove any loose flour from the sides and bottom. For machines that don't make gluten-free food, you can do this however you want. Let the rest be done by the machine. In my machine, the whole time is 3 hours.
5. If you don't want a big hole at the bottom, you can take the paddle out of the machine 31 minutes after my machine starts stirring. Also, you can top the bread with oatmeal or your favorite seeds if you want to. Use the backs of your moistened fingers to press the oatmeal and/or seeds into the dough.
6. If the kneading peddle is still in the bottom of the bread after it has been baked, take it out. Take on a wire rack and let cool for around 2 hours or until completely cool.
7. Use a knife with serrated edges, an electric meat/bread slicer with a serrated blade, or an electric knife with serrated edges to cut.
8. Use on toast or sandwiches. Slices that are left over can be frozen and then quickly thawed in the microwave or at room temperature.

36. JALAPENO CORN BREAD

Prep Time: 10 Minutes | Cook Time: 2-3 hours | Colling Time: 1 hour

Total Times: 3 hours 10 Minutes- 4 Hours 10 Minutes | Serving: 2 POUND

Ingredients

- 2 Tsp Crushed Red Pepper Flakes
- (~2 Tbsp.) Medium Jalapeño Peper, seeded & deveined
- 1 Tsp Cider Vinegar
- 1 Tbsp Xanthan Gum
- ½ Cup of(s) of Pumpkin Puree (not pumpkin pie filling)
- 2 Large Eggs, at room temperature, sligtly beaten
- 1 Active Dry Yeast Packet
- 1 Tsp Salt
- ¾ Cup of(s) Brown Rice Flour
- 2 Tsp Sugar
- ¾ Cup of(s) Lukewarm Water (85-95°F)
- ½ Cup of(s) Corn Starch
- 3 Tbsp Honey
- 2 ½ Tbsp Vegetable Oil
- ½ Cup of(s) Yellow Corn Meal
- ¾ Cup of(s) Tapioca Flour

Instructions

1. Combine rice and tapioca flour, xanthan gum, corn starch, corn meal, sugar, and Salt in a large bowl. Set aside.
2. Mix together eggs, water, pumpkin puree, honey, oil, and vinegar. Stir in Jalapeno peppers and red pepper flakes; pour the mixture into a bread pan.
3. Spoon flour mixture over top of liquids; sprinkle with yeast.
4. Put the bread pan in the baking chamber, close the lid, and plug the bread maker into the wall.
5. Select BASIC SETTING, 1.5 POUND. LOAF, MEDIUM CRUST. Then press START.
6. After the bread is done baking, put the bread from the pan and take it on a wire rack. Cool completely. Cut into slices to serve.

37. HERB & OLIVE LOAF BREAD

Prep Time: 15 Minutes

Cook Time: 30 Minutes

Total Times: 45 Minutes

Serving: 8

Ingredients

- ½ tsp salt
- ¼ cup of olive oil
- 2 tsp sugar
- 1-1/3 cup of warm water
- 3 ½ cups of Glutano Flour Mix
- 2 tsp Authentic Foods Dough Enhancer
- 2 eggs
- 2 tsp yeast
- 1 tsp apple cider vinegar
- ½ cup of Authentic Foods White Bread Mix

Instructions

1. Combine ingredients 1-6 and whisk thoroughly - you're done when it foams up.
2. Combine Glutano Flour Mix and Authentic Foods White Bread Mix in a bowl.
3. Place all wet ingredients (add the Salt) in the bread machine and mix thoroughly.
4. Start the bread machine and add the flour mix. Take Flour as needed so that the dough is firm enough NOT to fall back into the space created by the bread machine paddle.

38. ONION BREAD

Prep Time: 15 Minutes | Cook Time: 2-3 hours

Total Times: 2-3 hours 15 Minutes | Serving: 12 slice

Ingredients

- 1 1/2 Tsp – Salt
- 3 Cups of – Bread Flour (not all-purpose flour)
- 1 Cup of – Milk (lukewarm)
- 1 1/2 Tsp – Bread Machine Yeast
- 4 Tbsp – Unsalted Butter (softened)
- 1 Tbsp – White Granulated Sugar
- 1 Tbsp – Onion Powder
- 1/2 – Large Onion (diced & fried)

Instructions

1. The settings for a bread machine are Basic, Light Color, and 1.5 pound.
2. Cut the half onion into small pieces. Cook the diced onions in a small amount of butter/vegetable oil in a frying pan until they are golden brown.
3. Turn off the bread machine and take out the bread pan. First, pour the milk and butter that has been softened into the bread pan. Then, add the other ingredients. Place the yeast in the bread machine last. The yeast shouldn't touch the liquid, Salt, or hot onions that have been sautéed until the bread machine turns and the elements start to combine together. Make a small crater/ditch in the top of the Flour, and use this to hide the yeast from the Salt and other ingredients.
4. Take the bread pan with the ingredients back into the bread machine that has been turned off.
5. Turn on the breadmaker. Enter the right settings (basic, light color, and 1.5 pound) and press the "start" button.
6. When the bread is done baking in the bread machine, you should unplug it. Place the bread out of the oven and take it on a rack to cool. When you put the container out of the bread machine, use oven mitts because it will be very hot.
7. Don't forget to take out the mixing paddle if it's stuck in the bread after you take out the bread. Use oven mitts because the mixing paddle coming out of the bread machine will be very hot. Or, wait until the bread is completely cool and then take the paddle off the mixer.
8. Before using your bread machine, you should read the manufacturer's instructions carefully to use it effectively and safely.

39. CHEDDAR CHEESE BREAD

Prep Time: 10 Minutes | Cook Time: 4 Hours

Total Times: 4 Hours 10 Minutes | Serving: 14

Ingredients

Wet Ingredients:

- 1 ½ cups of water
- 2 Tbsp. Vegetable oil
- 3 eggs

Dry ingredients:

- 2 ¼ tsp. Active dry yeast
- ¼ cup of dry milk powder for a dairy-free option, try DariFree
- 1 tsp. salt
- 1 Tbsp. poppy seeds
- 2 Tbsp. white sugar
- 1 ½ dried dill weed
- 3 ½ tsp. xanthan gum
- 2 cups of white rice flour
- 1 cup of brown rice flour
- 1 ½ cups of shredded sharp Cheddar cheese. Try Daiya for a dairy-free option

Instructions

1. Mix the wet ingredients that are at room temperature together well in a medium bowl.
2. Take all of the dry ingredients together in a bowl. Make sure everything is mixed well with a wire whisk.
3. Put the wet ingredients in the pan of your bread machine first, then add the dry ingredients on top.
4. Select setting 3 – whole wheat setting – and press start.
5. For the first 5 minutes or so, keep a spatula handy to push the mixture down and make sure it's mixing well.
6. This setting should be about 4 hours – after it's done, remove the beautiful, long-awaited loaf from the pan, then cool it on a wire rack.

40. GARLIC PARMESAN BREAD

Prep Time: 20 Minutes | Cook Time: 4 Hour 5 Second | Additional Time: 20 minutes

Total Times: 4 Hours 40 Minutes 5 Second | Serving: 1 Loaf

Ingredients

- 2 tbsp of softened raw butter
- 2 1/2 tsp active dry yeast
- 2 tbsp of sugar
- 1 cup of room-temperature water
- 3 cups of gluten-free all-purpose Flour (you may use all-purpose flour)
- 1 1/2 tsp garlic salt
- 1/2 cup of grated Parmesan cheese
- 2 tsp dried onion flakes
- 1 large egg; lightly beaten

Instructions

1. In your bread machine, add all wet ingredients, water, eggs, and butter. Next, add your dry ingredients Flour, parmesan cheese, sugar, onion flakes, and garlic powder.
2. Most Importantly, make a small, hallow hole on top of your ingredients and fill with the yeast.
3. Furthermore, when preparing your Gluten Free Garlic/Parmesan Bread Machine, it is essential to add your yeast last.
4. Close the lid, and press the rapid bake cycle with the light crust setting.
5. Throughout the bread machine cycle, all your ingredients will be kneed, risen, and then baked.
6. My bread machine's total processing takes about three and a half hours, but checks with your user's manual on how long your bread will bake in the bread machine.
7. Once the cycle is complete, remove the bread immediately; now, it cools on a wire rack for about thirty minutes.
8. Slice the desired thickness with a serrated bread knife. Serve bread warm with butter or plain.
9. Store leftover bread in a zip-loc bag or bread bag for future use.

41. NUT FRERATAE LOW-CARB BREAD

Prep Time: 20 Minutes | Cook Time: 1 Hour 10 Minutes

Cooling Times: 1 Hour 30 Minutes | Total Times: 3 Hours

Serving: 15

Ingredients

- 1-1/3 cups of water 3 large eggs
- 4 tbsp butter melted and cooled (or ghee, margarine, or oil)
- 1-1/2 cups of golden flaxseed meal (170 g) (Bob's Red Mill)
- 1 cup of brown rice protein or pea protein or half of each** (118 g)(NOW Foods) 2 tbsp psyllium husk powder 16 g) (Vitacost)
- 2 tsp instant dry yeast SAF
- 1 tsp gluten-free baking powder Featherweight for corn-free
- 1-1/2 tsp guar gum for corn-free
- 1/4 tsp of monk fruit extract powder Lakanto, 1/2 tsp of salt ,: sugar-alcohol-free(or sugar-free substitute

Instructions

1. Add the water, eggs, and cooled melted butter to the bowl of your electric blender and combine on low speed just until combined. If making in the oven, add these ingredients to its bowl.
2. In a separate bowl, spatula together the flax seed meal, brown rice protein powder, yeast, baking powder, guar gum, Salt, and monk fruit extract powder; add to the liquid ingredients.
3. To cook in the oven, transfer to the prepared pan and set in a warm (80 – 90⁰F) environment for 1-1/2 hours or until it stops rising. (I use the bread proofer linked above. Alternatively, you can preheat your oven to the lowest or warm setting and then turn it off. Open the door to cool it down to about 84⁰Oil the top of the bread dough or a sheet of plastic wrap and cover with plastic wrap. Allow to rise in the oven with the door closed.) Bake for 1 hour 10 minutes. Tent with foil once the crust reaches your desired color. To make it in a machine, simply set it to gluten-free and press start or follow the manufactures instructions. Help stir in the very beginning, scraping down the sides.
4. Immediately take out from the pan and allow to cool for up to 2 hours or until it reaches room temperature.
5. Slice by hand using a serrated knife. Freeze leftovers in a zipper storage bag or air-tight container.

42. CHEESE LOAF BREAD

Prep Time: 5 Minutes | Cook Time: 2 Hours 10 Minutes

Resting Time:15 minutes | Total Times: 2 Hours 30 Minutes

Serving: 16 Slice

Ingredients

- 1 tsp Salt
- 3 cups of Tapioca Starch - 1 pack of 1Pound / 454g
- 3 Egg
- 1/2 tbsp Oregano - reserve
- 2 tsp Baking powder - reserve
- 1/2 cup of Parmesan cheese - grated - reserve - or more to taste
- 1/2 cup of Oil
- 1 cup of Milk
- 1 cup of Friulano cheese or Mozzarella cheese -shredded -reserve or more to taste

Instructions

1. Put the blade for kneading into the Bread Maker pan.
2. Put the ingredients in the bread pan in the order given in the recipe.
3. Before making gluten-free bread, the liquid ingredients must be whisked together in a separate bowl to make sure they mix well.
4. Place the bread pan carefully into the Bread Maker and close the lid gently.
5. Choose "Gluten-free" and then press the "Start" button.
6. Size and "Crust Color" can't be changed.
7. If your bread machine doesn't have a gluten-free setting, you should bake gluten-free bread on the Basic setting.
8. After pre-mixing for 6 minutes, use a Silicone Spatula to clean the pan of Flour. DO NOT take the pan away. KEEP it locked in the machine while you take the Flour off the sides.

43. PUMPERNICKEL BREAD

Prep Time: 25 Minutes | Cook Time: 1 Hour 10 Minutes

Total Times:1 Hour 35 Minutes | Serving: 20 Slice

Ingredients

For Sourdough Starter Activation:

- 1/3 cup of brown rice flour
- 1/4 cup of filtered water - (add 1 to 2 tbsp more if it's too thick)
- 1 cup of gluten-free sourdough starter - (previously made and refrigerated)

For The Dough:

- 2 tbsp maple sugar - or coconut sugar
- 1½ cup of buckwheat flour
- 2 tbsp pumpkin seeds - (ground like Flour)
- 1½ tbsp of pink Himalayan salt - or 1.5 tsp sea salt

- 2½ cups of filtered water - (+2 or 3 tbsp more if it's too thick)
- 1 tbsp coriander seeds - (ground like Flour)
- 2 tbsp sunflower seeds - (ground like Flour)
- 2 tbsp caraway seeds - (ground like Flour)
- 2 tbsp cacao powder - (optional – for a dark color) or carob powder
- 2 tbsp psyllium husk - not powder
- 1/2 cup of flax meal - (ground golden flax seeds)
- 2/3 cup of teff flour

Instructions

1. Use an electric coffee grinder to grind all of the seeds.
2. Activate The Gluten-Free Sourdough Starter:
3. If you just bought a dehydrated gluten-free sourdough starter, read the booklet that comes with it for instructions on how to activate it. This post will learn you how to make your own starter if you don't already have one.
4. Once the starter is working, put 1 cup of it in a large bowl. The others feed it and put it back in the fridge.
5. Then, combine 1/3 cup of brown rice flour and 1/4 cup of water with the gluten-free starter. Combine well. This step will turn on the cold dormant starter you just took out of the fridge.
6. If your starter is thin and watery, try using less water. Now the mixture sits in a warm place for 3–4 hours or until it's light and bubbly. If your house is cold, it could place up to 5 or 6 hours.

Form The Dough:

1. Add the water and psyllium husk once the starter is ready and working. Mix to blend. While you sift the rest of the Flour, the psyllium will grow in the water. Then, pour the Flour through a sieve into the same bowl. Blend everything together. The dough should look like brownie batter or a very thick pancake batter. There is no need to knead.

Bread Proofing:

1. It will help prevent sticking if you line the baking pan with parchment paper. I'm using an extendable baking tin. It doesn't have a bottom, so it's easy to take out of the oven when it's done. It moves easily in and out.
2. Put the dough in the pan and flatten it out. Top with caraway seeds.
3. Warp it with plastic wrap or a towel to place the moisture in, and let it rise in a warm place for about 4-5 hours (in the winter, it might take an extra hour or two).
4. It all depends on how hot your kitchen is. Depending on how cold your place is, it may take longer than that.

Bake The Bread:

1. Set the oven temperature to 425 F (220 C).
2. When you're ready to bake, take off the plastic wrap, cover with aluminum foil to keep out moisture (but don't touch it), lower the oven temperature to 380 F (200 C), and bake for 30 minutes.
3. Then, take the foil off. At this point, you can also take it out of the baking pan (so it cooks evenly on all sides) and bake it for another 40–50 minutes or until it's no longer soft when you touch it.
4. Then it cools completely before you touch it or cut it! More time is better. I usually slice it up the next day and freeze it.

44. RYE BREAD

Prep Time: 15 Minutes | Cook Time: 2-3 hours Minutes

Total Times: 2-3 hours 15 Minutes | Serving: 12 Slice

Ingredients

- 2 tbsp quinoa flour
- 3 tbsp of unsalted butter, room temperature, cut into ½-inch pieces
- ⅓ cup of cornstarch
- 2 large eggs, room temperature
- ⅓ cup of potato starch
- ¾ cup of brown rice flour
- ⅓ cup of sorghum flour
- 1½ tsp kosher Salt
- ¾ tsp cider vinegar
- 2¼ tsp yeast, active dry, instant, or bread machine
- ½ tsp gelatin
- 1½ cups of low-fat milk, room temperature
- ¾ tsp orange zest
- ¾ cup of garfava flour
- 1½ tbsp caraway seeds
- 2 tbsp light brown sugar, firmly packed
- 2 tsp xanthan gum

Instructions

1. Take all the ingredients in the bread pan with the kneading paddle in the order given. Secure the bread pan in the Cuisinart® Automatic Bread Maker. Press the menu button to select the Gluten Free program. Press Start/Stop to mix, rise and bake. While the dough is being mixed, take a rubber spatula or Silicone spatula to scrape the sides of the bread pan to make sure all of the ingredients are mixed in. When the cycle is done, Put the bread out of the bread pan and take it on a wire rack to cool completely.

45. POTATO BREAD

Prep Time: 15 Minutes | Cook Time: 1 hours 45Minutes

Total Times: 2 hours | Serving: 8-12

Ingredients

- 1 tsp xanthan gum (omit if your flour blend already includes it)
- 2 1/4 tsp instant yeast
- 1/4 tsp salt
- 2 large eggs, beaten
- 1 cup mashed potatoes
- 1 tbsp sugar
- 1/4 cup of sunflower oil
- 2 1/4 cups of gluten-free all-purpose flour
- 1 cup of warm water (between 105F to 115F)
- 2 tbsp psyllium husk powder

Instructions

1. Grease: Lightly oil an 8" x 4" loaf pan.
2. Stir Dry Ingredients: Sift the gluten-free all-purpose flour, instant yeast, sugar, salt, psyllium husk powder, and xanthan gum (if using it) into a large bowl. To combine, whisk thoroughly.
3. Blend: Using a high-speed blender, blend the eggs and mashed potatoes until you have a thick, creamy yellow mixture.
4. Transfer the mixture to a sizable mixing bowl and add the water and oil. A pale yellow liquid will result from thoroughly combining water and oil.
5. Create the dough: Combine the wet and dry ingredients in a bowl, stirring until a cohesive, sticky dough forms (the dough will appear fuzzy and be pretty wet, but that's the texture you want).
6. Transferring Dough to Pan: Transfer the dough to the prepared loaf pan, and smooth the dough's top with a wet spatula.
7. Cover the pan in a warm, draft-free area with a kitchen towel. Let the dough rise. The dough needs to grow for 40 to 50 minutes or until it has roughly doubled in size (I like to put the pan in the microwave with the power off).
8. Start the oven at 350°F and put the rack in the middle before the dough rises.
9. Bake it for 1 hour until the top is golden brown and touching the loaf makes a hollow sound.
10. Let Cool Before Slicing: After the loaf has cooled in the pan for 10 minutes, take it out and set it on a wire rack to finish cooling completely (at least 30 minutes) before slicing.

46. BLACK RUSSIAN BREAD

Prep Time: 15 Minutes | Cook Time: 1-2 hours

Total Times: 1-2 hour 15 Minutes | Serving: 1 Loaf

Ingredients
Wet ingredients:

- 1 tsp cider vinegar
- 3 large eggs, lightly beaten
- 2 tbsp molasses
- 3 tbsp olive oil
- 1 1/3 cups of water

Dry ingredients:

- 1/2 cup of tapioca starch
- 1 tbsp xanthan gum

- 1 1/2 tbsp cocoa
- 1 tsp instant coffee
- 1/2 cup of potato starch
- 2 tbsp caraway seeds
- 1/2 cup of non-fat dry milk
- 1 (0.2 Ounce) package (7g) or 2 1/4 tsp
- 1 1/2 tsp Salt
- 1/3 cup of rice bran
- 3 tbsp dark brown sugar, packed
- 2 cups of brown rice flour
- 1 tbsp egg replacer (optional)

Instructions

1. Check sure that everything is at room temperature. Take all the wet ingredients in a bowl with a whisk, then put the mixture into a baking pan. Take all of the dry ingredients in a separate bowl and whisk them together. Then, take the dry ingredients on top of the wet ingredients in the baking pan.
2. Choose the gluten-free cycle and turn on the machine. After the mixing starts, use a rubber spatula to work any unmixed ingredients into the dough. Stay near the edges and top of the batter to keep the kneading blade from getting in the way.
3. Take the pan out of the machine when the cycle is done. Now the bread stays in the pan for about 10 minutes, then flip the pan over and give it a gentle shake to take the bread out. Cool on a rack upright before slicing.

47. LEMON CHEESECAKE

Prep Time: 30 Minutes | Cook Time: 1-2 hours | Chilling Time: 3-4 hours

Colling Time: 1 hour | Total Times: 5-7 hours 30 Minutes | Serving: 8-12

Ingredients
For the dough:

- 50g melted butter
- 1 organic lemon
- 400g skyr/quark
- 30g cornstarch
- 80g sugar
- 1 vanilla pod

For the icing:

- 30g icing sugar
- 1 organic lemon

- 1 vanilla pod
- 150g cream cheese

Optional - toppings:

- coconut flakes
- pistachios
- fresh mint

Instructions

1. Preparation of the dough:
2. Butter the mixing bowl of the bread machine and put about 1 to 2 tbsp of gluten-free Flour in it. Turn the bowl back and forth to spread the Flour out evenly. Tap the gluten-free Flour to get rid of any extra. Take the mixing bowl in the refrigerator for half 1 hour.
3. Grate the organic lemon peel into small pieces and squeeze out the juice.
4. Get the vanilla bean out of the pod.
5. Corn starch and 2 tbsp of water should be mixed together until smooth.
6. Melt the butter in a pot, then cools for a few minutes.
7. Add the Skyr with sugar, the vanilla pulp that you scraped out, the grated lemon peel, and about 2 tsp of the lemon juice to the bread maker bowl.
8. Pour in the mix of water and starch.
9. Select the program "gluten-free cake" and let the breadmaker mix the dough. Remove the kneading blade after the mixing time is over.

10. Open the lid when the breadmaker is done baking the cake and the programmed time is up. Let the cake cool in the machine with the lid open for around half an hour. Then take the bowl away and let it cool at room temperature for another hour. Then take it in the refrigerator for 3 - 4 hours.
11. Once the cake has had time to cool, carefully loosen it all around with a silicone dough scraper and turn it over onto a wire rack or board.
12. To make the frosting, grate the organic lemon peel finely and squeeze out the juice.
13. Scrape out the vanilla pod.
14. Mix the cream cheese with 1/2 tsp of the lemon juice, the vanilla pulp that you scraped out, and the grated lemon peel until it is smooth. Mix in the powdered sugar.
15. Take a short break.
16. Spread onto the cold cheesecake with a spoon and optionally decorate.

48. BREAD RECIPE WITH CACAO AND FENNEL

Prep Time: 15 Minutes | Cook Time: 1-2 hours | Colling Time: 2 hours 15 Minutes

Total Times: 3-4 hours 30 Minutes | Serving: 8-12

Ingredients

- 2 tsp salt
- 4 tsp fennel seeds
- 2 tsp sugar
- 410-430ml lukewarm water
- 1 package (7g) dry yeast
- 60g walnuts
- 530g rice flour e.g. komeko brotgenuss
- 2 tsp cacao powder
- 1 tbsp psyllium husks

Instructions

1. With a whisk, mix the dry yeast, xylitol sugar, and about 100 ml of the warm water until the yeast is well dissolved. Then wait 5 to 10 minutes.
2. Use a mortar to make the fennel seeds as small as possible.
3. Make small pieces out of the walnuts.
4. With the kneading blade in place, place all of the dry ingredients into the bread pan of the bread machine.
5. Take the yeast mixture and the rest of the warm water into the bowl.
6. Choose "gluten-free bread" from the menu and press "start."
7. After the kneading time is up, you can take out the kneading blade if you want to.
8. If you need to, shape the dough again with a dough scraper and carefully cut the top of the dough. For a unique look, sprinkle a little rice flour on the dough.
9. You can also add 1 tbsp of gluten-free oat flakes and more chopped walnuts.
10. After the program is done, turn off the breadmaker but leave the bread inside for another 15 minutes so it can still get warm. Then put the bread out of the bread pan and put it on a board.
11. Let cool completely and wait at least 2 hours before cutting.

49. PIZZA DOUGH

Prep Time: 10 Minutes | Cook Time: 30 Minutes | Rising Time: 1 Hour

Total Times: 1 Minutes | Serving: 2

Ingredients

- 1 cup of brown rice flour 1 cup of white rice flour
- 1/2 cup of corn starch (or potato starch)
- 1/4 cup of extra virgin olive oil + more for brushing crust
- 1 1/2 cups of potato starch (or tapioca flour/starch)
- 1 Tbsp sugar
- 1 cup of buttermilk (or rice milk + 4 tsp apple cider vinegar and rested for 15 minutes) 1/4 cup of water, at room temperature
- 2 Tbsp instant yeast
- 1 tsp fine sea salt
- 1 Tbsp xanthan gum (or guar gum for corn-free) (Add 1/2 tsp. extra if not using tapioca flour/starch for a chewy texture.)
- 1 whole large egg 3 large egg whites, at room temperature

Instructions

1. Add ingredients to the bread machine bowl in the order listed above; help it along during the kneading by using a rubber spatula.
2. Place the bowl in the bread machine; close the lid; set to the dough setting; press start (my machine kneads for 30 minutes and rises for 1 hour). If using three 12-inch pizza pans or 2 12-by-17-inch baking/cookie sheets, preheat the oven to 425°F.
3. If you're using a pizza stone, preheat the oven with the stone inside to 500°F for crispy/direr crust and 450°F for a more traditional texture (though they'll both have a nice bottom crust).
4. Once the bread machine completes its cycles, remove the dough, then Cut it into 2 equal portions (3 for thinner crusts - makes thin crust); either with your hands,

distribute the dough evenly over the bottom of the pans (pre-dust with cornmeal, if desired).

5. If using a pizza stone, roll onto a lightly floured surface; roll around a rolling pin, and transfer to the preheated pizza stone.

6. If desired, brush the ends with olive oil for a darker crust. Pre-bake for 15 minutes on a baking sheet or about 8 minutes on a preheated stone.

7. Remove pan/stone from oven; top with your pizza toppings; return to oven and bake for approximately 12 minutes in a pan; 8 - 10 minutes on a rock, at 425°F (425°F for a crisper/darker crust).

8. Either repeat the above steps for the other dough or freeze it, wrapped in plastic wrap, and insert it into a freezer bag. If using a stone, preheat the stone for 10 minutes before proceeding with the second piece of dough.

50. SMOKED SALMON SALAD PIZZA

Prep Time: 10 Minutes | Cook Time: 15 Minutes

Total Times: 25 Minutes | Serving: 2 Pizza

Ingredients

Gluten Free Pizza Dough (makes 2 pizzas):

- 1/4 cup of (50g) teff flour
- 1 tsp. (3.5g) baking powder
- 2 cups of (296g) brown rice flour
- 1 Tbsp. (8.6g) active dry yeast
- 2 Tbsp. (26g) olive oil
- 1 tsp. (5.6g) salt
- 1-1/2 cups of (360mL) water
- 1 tsp. (1g) dried oregano
- 2 Tbsp. (40g) honey
- 1 Tbsp. (8g) xanthan gum
- 1/2 cup of (60g) tapioca flour
- 1/4 cup of (35g) corn starch
- 2 tsp. (7.4g) garlic powder

Balsamic Vinaigrette (for 1 pizza):

- 2 Tbsp. olive oil
- 1/2 tsp. ground black pepper
- 1/2 tsp. salt
- 1 Tbsp. balsamic vinegar
- 1/2 Tbsp. red wine vinegar

Topping (for 1 pizza):

- 1 Tbsp. chopped fresh dill
- 2.7 Ounce sliced smoked salmon (not seasoned)
- 1-2/3 cups of shredded mozzarella cheese (gluten free)
- 8-10 cherry tomatoes, cut in halves
- 4 Tbsp. ranch dressing (gluten free)
- 3 cups of spring mix salad
- 2 tsp. capers
- 3 Tbsp. thinly sliced onion

Instructions

1. Mix the brown rice flour, teff flour, tapioca flour, corn starch, xanthan gum, and baking powder in a large bowl with a whisk.
2. Ensure the kneading blade(s) are correctly attached, then put the water, olive oil, and honey in the baking pan. Add the flour mixture from step 1, salt, garlic powder, and dried oregano, to the baking pan. Make a hole in the flour with a Tiny spoon and put the yeast there. Make sure the yeast doesn't get in contact with the liquid and salt.
3. Set the BB-PAC20 model to the regular DOUGH course or the BB-CEC20 model to the introductory dough course, and then press START.
4. When the class is over,
5. Take out the dough from the pan and transfer it to a surface lightly dusted with flour. Half the dough and roll each half into a smooth ball. Cover the balls with wet paper towels and let them rest for 30 minutes.
6. Turn the oven on to 375°F. Put parchment paper on a pizza pan and grease it with 1 tbsp of olive oil, which is out of the list of ingredients. Wet your hands with water, take one piece of dough, and flatten it into a 10" circle with slightly raised edges. Make a small hole in the dough with a fork. 15 minutes in an oven that has already been turned on. The dough must not be allowed to rise too much; it is best to bake the second pizza the same day.
7. While the pizza is in the oven, get the topping ready. All ingredients for balsamic vinaigrette should be mixed in a large bowl. Mix the dressing well with the spring mix salad, tomatoes, onions, and capers.
8. When the crust is done, shredded mozzarella cheese should be evenly distributed on top before baking.
9. Remove the crust from the dish and carefully transfer it onto a cutting board. Place the salad already mixed on top and top it with the smoked salmon and dill. Drizzle with ranch dressing. Cut it up and serve it hot.

51. PIZZA CRUST

Prep Time: 2 Hour | Cook Time: 45 Minutes

Total Times: 2 Hour 45 Minutes | Serving: 2 Pizza

Ingredients

Wet Ingredients:

- 1/2 cup of olive or grapeseed oil
- 3 large eggs
- 1 cup of milk
- 1/2 cup of water

Dry Ingredients:

- More cornstarch, for dusting
- 2 cups of rice flour or gluten free oat flour
- 1/2 cup of potato starch
- 3 tsp xanthan gum
- 1/2 cup of sugar
- 1 tsp salt
- 2 tbsp yeast
- 1 cup of cornstarch

Instructions

1. Mix the wet ingredients in a separate bowl, then pour them into the pan of the bread machine. Mix the dry ingredients in the bowl. Add to pan.
2. Put the bread-maker pan in the bread-maker and choose your regular cycle. When the "knead" part of this cycle is done, which takes about an hour, take the pan out of the bread machine.
3. While the dough is still being worked, grease two large pizza pans and sprinkle cornstarch on a clean surface.
4. Dump the dough and keep it on the floured surface. Knead it for a few minutes. Slice the dough into two equal portions, and place each half on separate pans.
5. Let the dough rise for an hour. Prepare the toppings while the dough rises.
6. When the dough has finished rising, add toppings and put the pizzas in the oven.
7. Cook it for around 45 minutes at 350 degrees F or until the crust becomes golden brown.

52. PIZZA RECIPE

Prep Time: 30 Minutes | Cook Time: 50 Minutes

Total Times: 1 Hour 20 Minutes | Serving: 1 Pizza

Ingredients
Dough:

- 20g potato starch
- 1 packet dry yeast
- 1/2 tbsp xanten
- 1 tbsp psyllium husks
- 1 tbsp baking powder
- 110g teff flour and 1 tsp salt
- 30g cornstarch
- 100g chickpea flour
- 170ml lukewarm water
- 2 tbsp xylitol
- 1 tbsp dried herbs

Topping:

- pinch of pepper
- a hand full of olives
- 6 cocktail tomatoes
- pinch of salt
- 50g tomato puree
- 50g strained tomatoes
- 80g vegan fresh cheese
- 1 tsp sweetener of choice
- 1 tbsp dried basil

Instructions

1. Mix 50 ml of warm water with the dry yeast and xylitol.
2. Pour the ingredients (dry) into the Croustina bread pan one at a time, and use a spatula to roughly mix them together.
3. Add the yeast mixture along with the remainder of the lukewarm water. Use the dough scraper to mix the ingredients together in a rough way.
4. Close the routine and choose Program 14 for gluten-free bread.
5. Let the Croustina do its thing. After the dough has been kneaded, it rests in the chosen program. After 30 minutes of cooking time, the program can be turned off.
6. Remove the dough from the bowl and repeat the kneading process on a surface that has been dusted with flour.
7. Preheat the oven to around 200°C.
8. Shape the mass into two pizzas. The pizzas should be put on a baking sheet.
9. Cut the cocktail tomatoes into fourths. Make thin slices of the olives.
10. Mix the strained tomatoes, tomato puree, sliced olives, your choice of sweetener, salt, and pepper to make a tomato sauce, which you then spread on the pizzas.
11. Fresh tomatoes are cut and go on top.Put chunks of fresh vegan cheese on the pizza.
12. Bake it for 20 minutes, depending on how thick the dough is and what texture you want.

53. SANDWICH BREAD

Prep Time: 15 Minutes | Cook Time: 40 Minutes

Total Times: 55 Minutes | Serving: 12

Ingredients

- 1 tsp guar gum
- 1 Tbsp xanthan gum
- 3 cups of gluten-free all-purpose baking flour
- 1 tsp cider vinegar or lemon juice
- 2 Tbsp sugar
- 1/4 cup of vegetable oil
- 3/4 cup of whole egg (must measure 3/4 cups)
- 1 1/2 cups of warm milk (cow, rice, soy, or nut)
- 3/4 tsp sea salt
- 2 tsp active dry yeast
- 3/4 tsp lecithin granules (plain soy)
- 1 Tbsp potato flour

Instructions

1. Ensure that everything is at room temperature.
2. Whisk the liquids together until they are very smooth. Pour the liquids into the bread pan.
3. Whisk the dry ingredients, except the yeast, in a separate bowl until they are well mixed. The dry ingredients go on top of the wet ingredients.
4. In the middle of the dry ingredients, make a small well and put the yeast in it.
5. Pick the Gluten-Free Cycle. Hit "Start." When the bread is done, take it out of the bread machine and carefully take the kneading paddle off the bottom of the loaf.
6. Let it cool for 10 minutes before you use a bread knife to cut it.

54. SORGHUM-MILLET SANDWICH BREAD

Prep Time: 10 Minutes | Cook Time: 1 Hour 30 Minutes | Inactive Time: 5 Minuites

Total Times: Minutes | Serving: 14 Slice

Ingredients

- 3 tbsps honey
- 1/4 cup of softened butter
- 2 2/3 tsps instant yeast
- 2/3 cup of millet flour
- 1 2/3 tsps salt
- 2/3 cup of potato starch
- 2 cups of sorghum flour
- 2/3 cup of tapioca starch
- 2/3 tsp lemon juice (or cider vinegar)
- 1 1/3 cups of warm water
- 2 2/3 tsps xanthan gum
- 3 large eggs (lightly beaten)

Instructions

1. Mix together the flours, starches, gum, salt, and yeast in a large bowl.
2. Add the dry and wet ingredients (EXCEPT the butter) to the bread pan according to the manufacturer's directions.
3. Choose the "Quick" cycle (2 pounds) and press the "Start" button.
4. When all the ingredients are mixed, use a spatula to scrape the sides of the bread pan and add the butter. (The dough should be thick, like muffin batter. If it's too thin, add 1 tbsp of warm water or flour.)
5. When the kneading cycle is done, take out the paddles and use a wet spatula to smooth the top of the dough.
6. When bread is done baking, after 30 minutes of cooling on a wire rack, cut it into slices using a serrated knife.

55. SANDWICH BREAD AND DINNER ROLLS

Prep Time: 15 Minutes | Cook Time: 60 Minutes | Additional Time: 30 Minuites

Total Times: 1 Hour 45 Minutes | Serving: 2 POUND Loaf

Ingredients

Dry Ingredients:

- 3 cups of (405 gr)gfJules® All-Purpose Gluten-Free Flour
- 1/4 cup of (26 gr) flax seed meal (or GF buckwheat; millet; sorghum, OR brown rice flour)
- 1/4 cup of dry milk powder, dairy or non-dairy (e.g. Coconut Milk Powder) {OR gluten free vanilla pudding mix OR protein powder}
- 1/2 tsp. baking soda
- 2 tsp. baking powder
- 1 tsp. sea salt

PLUS these Liquid:

- 1 Tbs. rapid rise or bread machine yeast, gluten-free
- 1/4 cup of extra virgin olive oil
- 1 1/4 cup of room temperature liquid: EITHER sparkling water, club soda, ginger ale or gluten free beer, milk of choice (not skim), OR plain yogurt*
- 2 large eggs (or 2 Tbs. flax seed meal steeped for 10 minutes in 6 Tbs. hot water) or other egg substitute
- 1 tsp. apple cider vinegar
- 2 Tbs. honey, agave nectar, date syrup OR coconut palm nectar

Toppings (optional):

- 1 Tbs. flaxseeds or sesame seeds, herbs or certified gluten free purity protocol oats
- 1 Tbs. coarse sea salt

Instructions

1. Using a breadmaker to bake bread is easy. There are three steps: It's best to start with the liquids, add the dry ingredients, and finally, the yeast.

2. Allow all liquids to come to room temperature, if possible, before placing them in the machine. Mix the yolks and whites with a whisk before putting them in the bread machine with the other liquids. Let the flax seed meal soak in water for 10 minutes before adding it. Whisk the dry ingredients together, then put them on top of the liquids in the pan. Make sure a small well with your finger in the midpoint of the dry ingredients and pour in the yeast.

3. Choose either the gluten-free bread setting or a 2 pound loaf with only one rise cycle and no punch-down. Close the bread machine's lid and let it do the rest.

4. During the mixing cycle, check on the dough to ensure the flour around the edges is mixed in. If not, use a rubber spatula to help the mixture reach the pan's edges and corners.

5. When the machine is finished mixing, smooth the top with a rubber spatula and add any toppings you want. Close the lid once more to bake.

6. Once the bake cycle is done, use a bread baking thermometer to check the temperature inside the loaf before taking it out of the pan. It should be at least 205o F. If it hasn't reached that temperature yet, add another 5–10 minutes of baking time to your bread machine or put the pan in a regular oven set to 350o F (static) and check the temperature every five minutes.

56. HALLOWEEN SANDWICH COOKIES

Prep Time: 60 Minutes | Cook Time: 30 Minutes

Total Times: 1 Hour 30 Minutes | Serving: 6

Ingredients

For the dough:

- 30g liquid coconut oil
- 1 tsp baking powder
- 1 pinch of turmeric
- 60g coconut blossom sugar
- 120g ground almonds
- 1 tsp pumpkin spice
- 160g rice flour (e.g. KOMEKO Knusperlust)
- 70g maple syrup
- 30g carrot and turmeric juice
- 25g plant-based milk

For the filling:

- 250g dark chocolate
- 3 tbsp plant-based milk
- 1 tsp pumpkin spice
- 1 vanilla pod

Additionally:

- 1 walnut-sized piece of turmeric
- 3-4 carrots
- 150g powdered sugar
- 1-2 tsp lemon juice

Instructions

1. First, make the juice by putting carrots and turmeric in the slow juicer and making juice out of them.
2. Heat the top and bottom of the oven to 175 degrees.
3. Program 15 of Croustina tells you to knead the dough. Mix the dry parts of the dough. Mix the liquid coconut oil, maple syrup, plant-based milk, carrot, and turmeric juice, and then add them to the dry ingredients.
4. Then, cut the dough into three pieces and roll each out to a thickness of about 0.5 cm on a floured surface. Cut out circles and put them all over a baking sheet. Bake the biscuits for 6–8 minutes or until the tops are golden brown. Then cool .
5. Melt the chocolate for the center. Throw in the spices. Stir the plant-based milk into the melted chocolate until the mixture gets thicker. Then put the mixture in the fridge for another 20 to 30 minutes, until it is a bit firmer but still creamy. Pour some chocolate filling into a piping bag and spread it on one of the cookies. Top with another cookie and press down. Let it sit for 30 minutes.
6. Mix powdered sugar and lemon juice to make icing sugar. It should stick together. Put a small amount of icing sugar on top of the biscuit.
7. Spider webs can decorate the biscuits. Use black sugar letters or food-colored liquid dark chocolate to do this. Draw three circles on icing. Use a toothpick to draw spider web lines from the circles. Let biscuits dry for 30 minutes.

57. POLENTA WITH MUSHROOMS

Prep Time: 20 Minutes | Cook Time: 50 Minutes

Total Times: 1 Hour 10 Minutes | Serving: 12 Slice

Ingredients

For the polenta:

- 1l lukewarm or warm water
- 200g organic corn flour
- 3g salt

For the mushroom sauce:

- 1 tbsp of lentil or classic tamari
- 1 bay leaf
- 15g spring onions

- 6-8 leaves fresh sage
- 2g kuzu arrowroot
- 15g vegetable stock
- 1 clove of garlic
- 30ml homemade almond milk
- 30g extra virgin olive oil
- salt to taste
- 300g cleaned mixed mushrooms
- 2g chopped rosemary

Instructions

1. Start with lukewarm water (not cold!), then put the polenta flour and salt in the breadmaker. Choose the compotes or jams program.
2. In the meantime, slice or cube the mushrooms and cut the spring onions into long strips.
3. Heat the oil in a pan that won't stick, then add the garlic, spring onion, and bay leaf. Add the mushrooms and salt when the garlic is simmering and cook for 8 to 10 minutes. Add the sage and salt to the pan, stir, and cook for one more minute.
4. In a separate bowl, whisk the arrowroot or kudzu, nondairy milk, and tamari together, making sure there are no lumps.
5. Pour them in to a pan with the mushrooms and let it simmer for 1 to 2 minutes. Reduce until the consistency you want is reached. Use a wooden spoon to mix, and if you need to, add the stock.
6. Before 1 or 2 minuites cooking done add the chopped rosemary.
7. Take out the garlic and bay leaf, put the hot polenta on a wooden cutting board, and serve with the mushroom sauce.

58. MULTI-GRAIN SANDWICH BREAD

Prep Time: 5 Minutes | Cook Time: 1 Hour 30 Minutes

Total Times: 1 Hour 35 Minutes | Serving: 16 Slice

Ingredients

- 1 cup of potato starch
- 1/ 1/4 tsp sea salt
- Sesame and/or caraway seeds
- 1/2 cup of GF Millet Flour
- 1 1/4 cups of warm liquid
- Pinch of sugar for the yeast
- 1/3 cup of Bob's Red Mill Gluten-Free Cornmeal
- 2 tsp xanthan gum

- 3 tbsp honey or raw agave nectar
- 2/3 cup of sorghum flour
- 1/2 tsp mild tasting rice vinegar (or lemon juice)
- 1 packet rapid or instant dry yeast or 2 1/4 tsp
- Ener-G Egg Replacer for 2 eggs
- 4 tbsp extra virgin olive oil

Instructions

1. To test the yeast, sprinkle it into warm water and add a little sugar.
2. Mix the dry things with a whisk. Mix the yeast left out to rise with olive oil, honey, rice vinegar (or lemon juice), and salt in a separate bowl. Set your machine to make 1.5 loaves with a medium crust. I used the gluten-free cycle on the Breadman. A rapid rise cycle will also work if you don't have a gluten-free process.
3. After mixing for a minute or two, open the machine and use a soft spatula to scrape down the main sides of the pan to help blend in the flour. I had to do this twice. Before the Rise cycle, when the mixing and kneading cycle was done, I took out the paddle and pressed and smoothed the top of the dough with wet fingers to make it look more even. I put a generous tbsp of sesame seeds on top.
4. When the machine beeped "done," it was done. I looked at the loaf to see if it was done well. This is accomplished by lightly pressing on the side. If it appears soft or gives too much, I add another 5 to 10 minutes of baking time (Select Bake only).
5. When the loaf seems done, remove it from the hot machine and put it on a wire rack. Turn it on its side and wiggle it out when it cools. It will steam and get too wet if you don't do this. Thump the loaf on a wire rack to see if it's done. The thump test shows if it's finished or not. When you tap on it, its sound hollow.
6. If it's not done, put the loaf directly on the middle rack of the oven and raise the temperature to 350oF. Check it after 10 minutes of baking. It should sound hollow when tapped and feel solid. Wire racks should cool the loaf. Cut with a toothed knife.

59. ROSEMARY SANDWICH BREAD

Prep Time: 15 Minutes | Cook Time: 1 Hour 30 Minutes | Rise Time: 40 Minuite

Total Times: 2 Hour 25 Minutes | Serving: 12 slice

Ingredients

- 1/4 cup of light extra virgin olive oil or oil of choice
- 3/4 cup of gluten-free oat flour or 2/3 cup of sorghum flour
- 1-1/2 cups of + 2 tbsp water
- 2/3 cup of brown rice flour
- 4 tsp freshly minced rosemary or 1 tbsp dry
- 1/2 cup of, at room temperature (or 6 tbsp liquid from a can of cannellini beans + 3 tbsp butter or DF margarine)

- 1 tsp apple cider vinegar
- 2 tbsp apple pectin powder
- 1/4 cup of cornstarch or tapioca flour/starch
- 1-1/4 cups of + 2 tbsp potato starch
- 2 tbsp honey or a gave or sugar
- 1/4 cup of non-fat instant dry milk
- 1 tbsp xanthan gum or guar gum for corn-free
- 3 large eggs
- 1 tsp salt

Instructions

1. Keep wet ingredients in a bowl of your bread maker; set aside.
2. Put the dry ingredients in a different bowl, mix them together, and then sprinkle them over the wet ingredients.
3. Utilize a bread machine equipped with a gluten-free setting and carefully adhere to the instructions provided by the manufacturer. (I use setting number 10 for gluten free.) This batter needs a little help in mixing at the start of the mixnig cycle. Using a silicone spatula, scrape the bottom and sides of the bread machine bowl to get the dough going. Then, allow the bread machine to do the rest.
4. In my machine, after 31 minutes of mixing, I start the machine and using a silicone spatula, I lift the dough up on one side and remove the mixing paddle. This prevents a really large hole in the bottom of the bread. A smaller one may remain. Then, allow the bread machine do the rest. Total time, 3 hours in the Breadman machine.
5. Once baked, remove the kneading paddle, if not already done.
6. Move the loaf to a wire rack, allowing it to cool entirely for approximately 2 hours.
7. Slice using an electric slicer, electric knife, or serrated knife.
8. Use for sandwiches, toast, or French toast. Freeze leftover slices and thaw as needed in the microwave on reheat for a few seconds, turning the bread over halfway through. Do not overheat or the bread will become rubbery as with most baked goods in the microwave.

60. CORN BREAD

Prep Time: 10 Minutes | Cook Time: 20 Minutes

Total Times: 30 Minutes | Serving: 8

Ingredients

- 1 tsp. salt
- 1 egg
- Add water to get a batter-like consistency up to one cup
- 2 cups of cornmeal (Make sure it's the granular cornmeal and not a cornmeal or corn mix that has been ground to a flourlike consistency)
- 4 tbsp. butter
- 1 ½ cups of plain yogurt or sour cream or buttermilk or milk. You can also combine them any way you like to total 1 ½ cups
-
- 1 tsp. baking soda
- 4 tbsp. honey
- 2 tsp. baking powder

Instructions

1. Put the ingredients in the bread pan of the bread machine in the order shown. Choose either "cake bread" or "batter bread." If your machine doesn't have one, choose the dough setting, but take the batter out before the dough setting starts the rising cycle. If you have one, you could also use a setting for pizza or pasta dough. There is no rise cycle for these two settings.
2. Set the oven temperature to 400° F/205° C.
3. Spread a lot of butter on a 12x12-inch glass baking dish, then pour the batter in. When the oven gets perfect temperature is ready, put the dish on the middle rack and bake for 15 to 20 minutes. After 15 minutes, test the center of the cornbread with a toothpick. When it becomes dry, Remove it from the oven and let it sit for about 10 minutes. If not, give it five more minutes. Cut it up and serve.

61. NO YEAST BREAD

Prep Time: 20 Minutes | Cook Time: 60 Minutes

Total Times: 1 Hour Minutes | Serving: 1 Loaf

Ingredients

Dry Ingredients:

- 3 cups of (405 gr) gfJules™ All-Purpose Gluten-Free Flour
- 1/2 tsp. baking soda
- 1 fJules™ Original Gluten Free Bread Mix
- 2 tsp. baking powder
- 1 tsp. sea salt
- 1/4 cup of flax seed meal (or GF buckwheat; millet; sorghum or brown rice flour)
- 1/4 cup of dry milk powder, dairy or non-dairy (e.g. Coconut Milk Powder) OR almond meal

Liquids for all:

- 2 Tbs. honey, agave nectar or coconut palm nectar (optional)
- 2 large eggs (OR 2 Tbs. flax seed meal steeped for 10 minutes in 6 Tbs. hot water)

- 1 tsp. apple cider vinegar (only if not using my gfJules™ Bread Mix)
- 1/4 cup of extra virgin olive oil
- 1 1/4 cup of club soda or sparkling water {with UPDATED Bread Mix may use regular water}

Plus for all:

- 1 Tbs. lemon juice
- 2 1/2 tsp. additional baking soda

Optional Toppings:

- 1 Tbs. crushed nuts, flaxseeds or sesame seeds (optional)
- 1 Tbs. coarse sea salt (optional)

Instructions

1. Set the oven temperature to 325o F (convection) or 350o F (static).
2. From Scratch: Mix the GF flours, milk powder, 1/2 tsp baking soda, 2 tsp baking powder, and 1 tsp salt in a large bowl.
3. Mix the honey (if you're using it), club soda, apple cider vinegar (not needed if you're using my bread mix), oil, egg, and honey (if you're using it) in the large bowl of a stand mixer. Pour the dry ingredient mix or bread mix packet into the wet bowl slowly, but don't add the yeast packet that comes with the bread mix.
4. Use a wooden spoon or the paddle attachment on a stand mixer to start mixing. Add the last bit of lemon juice and baking soda to the bowl before thoroughly mixing. When added together, the mixture should bubble up. If it doesn't, your baking soda isn't fresh enough. Once everything is mixed in, beat well for another minute or two.
5. Put the dough in an oiled 8.5 x 4 or larger bread pan. Use a dark metal pan if you like a darker crust on your bread. Use a lighter, shiny metal or glass pan if you want a more delicate crust.
6. Wet a large knife with a serrated edge and make two or three significant cuts about 1/2 inch deep in the top of the bread by rocking the blade back and forth in the wet dough. This will leave a mark. These cuts will make it easy for the bread to rise and open up.
7. This recipe's baking soda, baking powder, lemon juice, and club soda make the bread rise high. This can make the top crust look weird and hilly, but making these cuts before baking can help it look more even. No matter what the top crust looks like, the bread tastes great, so don't worry.
8. Smooth the top, add any toppings, and bake for about 60 minutes, or until the crust is nicely browned and a cake tester or skewer inserted into the center of the loaf comes out clean (the internal temperature should reach 205-210o F). After 50 minutes of baking, check the temperature to ensure the bread doesn't get too done.
9. Put on a rack to cool. After 15 minutes, carefully remove it from the loaf pan and let it cool before cutting it.
10. Once it's completely cool, put it in a bag with a zip-top on the counter. You can also cut and freeze it in a freezer bag with wax paper between the pieces. Do not put it in the fridge.

62. BEER BREAD

Prep Time: 45 Minutes | Cook Time: 35 Minutes

Total Times: 1 Hour 20 Minutes | Serving: 1 Loaf

Ingredients

Dry Ingredients:

- MIssing
- 1 gfJules Sandwich Bread Mix

OR:

- 3 cups of gfJules™ All Purpose Flour (405 grams)
- 1 tsp. sea salt (5 grams)
- 1/4 cup of dry milk powder/non-dairy milk powder (coconut milk powder 27 grams) OR almond meal (44 grams) OR plain GF potato flakes (16 grams)
- 1 Tbs. granulated cane sugar (16 grams)

PLUS:

- 3 Tbs. olive oil
- 2 Tbs. honey or agave nectar
- 2 1/4 tsp. (one packet) rapid rise or bread machine yeast
- 1 tsp. apple cider vinegar
- 10 ounce gluten free beer (I especially like Green's or Glutenberg in this recipe) or sparkling water, club soda or ginger ale – room temperature
- 3 large eggs — room temperature or substitute**
- sesame seeds, poppy seeds or other topping of choice (optional)

Instructions

- Prepare a standard loaf pan at least 9x5 inches by greasing it well. Set aside.
- Whisk the eggs, oil, apple cider vinegar, and honey in a large bowl.
- In another bowl, whisk all the dry ingredients (flour, salt, milk powder, and sugar) except for the yeast. When the mixer is on low speed, add the dry ingredients step by step to the wet ingredients.
- Keep beating as you slowly pour the beer in to mix. When everything is mixed, add the yeast. Make sure to beat the batter until it is completely smooth. Then, speed up the mixer and continue to beat for 4 minutes.
- To prepare, coat the pan with grease and pour only half of the batter.
- Cover with oiled wax paper or parchment paper and rise it in a warm, moist place for at least 30 minutes (an oven preheated to 200 F and then turned off with a bowl of water in the oven is a good option). Don't let the bread rise over the edge of the pan. If you do, it will get too big to stay up and may fall apart when it cools.
- After the bread has risen, brush it lightly with oil to help it brown, and add any toppings.
- Set the oven's temperature to 375o F (static) or 350o F (convection). About 35 minutes is enough time to bake. The temperature inside the bread should be between 205 and 210o F. The bread should have a higher rise than the top of the pan and a golden crust for optimal results.
- Take it from the pan and cool it there for 15 minutes. Lay it on one side, then the other, to help it stay in place as it cools. After baking, remove the loaf from the pan and put it on a wire rack for cooling it well.
- Don't cut until it's totally cool. Put your bread in a bag with a zip-top and leave it on the counter. To prevent it from drying out, avoid storing it in the refrigerator.

63. BREAD WITH BACON & OLIVES

Prep Time: 25 Minutes | Cook Time: 1 Hour 5Minutes

Total Times: 1 Hour 30 Minutes | Serving: 6

Ingredients

- 350ml water
- 1 tbsp honey
- 450g gluten free flour
- 1 tsp cider vinegar
- 2 medium eggs
- 1 tsp salt
- 100g cooked lean bacon
- 50g pitted black olives
- 1 tbsp oil
- 1 ½ tsp yeast

Instructions

1. In the order given, put all the ingredients into the bread pan.
2. Set your Croustina Breadmaker to make bread without gluten and with a dark crust.
3. When the bake time end, take out the bread and let it cool before cutting it.

64. SWEET POTATO CORNBREAD WITH WALNUTS

Prep Time: 30 Minutes | Cook Time: 1 Hour 55 Minutes

Total Times: 2 Hour 25 Minutes | Serving:

Ingredients

- 50g cranberries
- 1 tbsp salt
- 1 sachet dry yeast
- 1 tbsp salt
- 350g flour
- 250g polenta
- 100g almonds
- 1 sweet potato
- 80g crème fraîche
- 50ml olive oil
- 50g walnut kernels

Instructions

1. Peel the sweet potato and cut them into small pieces, and boil it in 200 ml of salted boiling water for about 10 minutes. Drain the sweet potato cubes well after pouring off the water. Then use the Panasonic high-performance mixer (function: puree) to blend the ingredients with olive oil until smooth.
2. In the pan of the Panasonic bread maker, combine the crème fraiche, 300 ml of water, ground almonds, polenta, flour, walnuts, cranberries, salt, and sweet potato puree. To the yeast distributor, add the dry yeast. The bread should be baked in the Panasonic bread machine on program 19/medium tan.
3. We also suggest a tasty dip made of curd and herbs.

65.SOURDOUGH ONION BREAD WITH PUMPKIN

Prep Time: 15 Minutes | Cook Time: 6 Hour

Total Times: 6 Hour 15 Minutes | Serving: 10

Ingredients

- 260ml water
- 2 onions
- 80g sourdough starter
- 1g yeast
- 8g salt
- 2 tbsp olive oil
- 310g spelt flour
- 90g wholemeal spelt flour
- 60g hokkaido pumpkin

Instructions

1. Take the bread maker pan out of the bread machine and add 260ml of water and the flour. Put the bread pan back in the machine, choose Menu 7 from the menu, and press the "Start" button. After about an hour, the machine will beep, letting you know that you can add the other ingredients.
2. chop the onions finally and add them to olive oil in a pan. Fry them for 40 minutes on low to medium heat until it becomes golden brown color. (Don't forget to stir the onions every now and then.) When the onions are done, keep them aside. Grate the pumpkin into small pieces and set them aside.
3. When the machine beeps, add the sourdough starter, salt, yeast, and vegetables to the breadmaker and press start again to continue the program.

66. BAGUETTES RECIPE

Prep Time: 30 Minutes | Cook Time: 10 Minutes

Total Times: 40 Minutes | Serving: 6

Ingredients

- 225ml water
- 10g dried rice sourdough
- 80g KOMEKO rice flour
- 60g buckwheat flour
- 2 tsp carob flour
- 1tbsp psyllium husk powder
- 1 tbsp cider vinegar
- 1 tsp salt
- 1 tsp cane sugar
- 1 tbsp rapeseed oil
- ½ cube fresh yeast
- 80g potato starch

Instructions

1. Choose program 14 (Gluten-free Bread) and press the "Start" button. Put the water, yeast, and sugar into the breadmaker's pan and let it sit for 5 minutes or more. Add the other ingredients and put the lid back on. Knead the dough, then set it aside for 20 minutes so it can rise. Stop the program once the dough has doubled and turn it onto a rice-floured work surface.
2. Cut the dough into half size and shape them into a baguette. Put the loaves in the nonstick grill pan, the wire rack in the cold microwave oven, and the pan on top of the rack. Set the temperature to 220 °C and choose the convection program (preheating). When the preheating is done, open the door for a moment and then close it right away. Then, set the bread machine a timer for 10 minutes and bake the baguettes until they are done.
3. Take the baguettes out of the microwave and let them cool down.

67. CRANBERRY, PUMPKIN & PECAN BREAD

Prep Time: 10 Minutes | Cook Time: 50 Minutes

Total Times: 1 Hour | Serving: 24

Ingredients

- 1/2 tsp all spice
- 50g dried cranberries
- 1 tsp salt
- 500g strong white flour
- 50g toasted pecans
- 1 tsp yeast
- 320ml water
- 100g roasted pumpkin or butternut squash
- 1/2 tsp nutmeg
- 1 tbsp olive oil
- 1/2 tsp ground ginger
- 1/2 tsp cinnamon
- 1 tbsp sugar

Instructions

1. Put everything but the pecans in the bread pan in the order listed above.
2. If you have a dispenser for raisins and nuts, put the pecans in it. If you don't, set them aside to add to the beep.
3. Set the bread machine to large size Basic Raisin Bake (4 hours).

68. SOURDOUGH RYE BREAD

Prep Time: 10Minutes | Cook Time: 45 Minutes | Additional Time: 10 Hour

Total Times: 10 Hour 55 Minutes | Serving: 1 Loaf

Ingredients

Wet ingredients:

- 3/4 cup of Gluten Free Sourdough Starter
- 3/4 cup of ricotta cheese (whole, part skim, or non-fat)
- 1/4 cup of vegetable oil
- 1 cup of water
- 3 large eggs
- 1 tsp cider vinegar
- 1/4 cup of molasses

Dry ingredients:

- 3 1/2 tsp xanthan gum
- 1 1/2 tsp salt
- 2/3 cup of potato starch
- 1/2 cup of dry milk powder
- 1/3 cup of tapioca flour
- 1 tbsp caraway seeds
- 2 tsp instant coffee
- 2 cups of white rice flour

Instructions

1. Put everything but the pecans in the bread pan in the order listed above.
2. If you have a dispenser for raisins and nuts, put the pecans in it. If you don't, set them aside to add to the beep.
3. Set the bread machine to a large-size Basic Raisin Bake (4 hours).

69.APPLE WALNUTS CAKE

Prep Time: 15 Minutes | Cook Time: 30 Minutes

Total Times: 45 Minutes | Serving: 15

Ingredients

- 1/3 cup of (46g) potato starch
- 3 large eggs, beaten
- 2 tsp. (7.0g) baking powder
- 1 tsp. (5.6g) salt
- 1 tsp. (5.3g) baking soda
- 3 Tbsp. (21g) tapioca flour
- 3/4 cup of (162g) vegetable oil
- 3 tsp. (6.0g) ground cinnamon
- 1 tsp. (2.1g) ground nutmeg
- 1 cup of (198g) sugar
- 1 tsp. (2.5g) xanthan gum
- 1-1/4 cups of (185g) brown rice flour
- When beeps sound, add:
- 1/2 cup of (55g) chopped walnuts
- 2 cups of (196g) fresh apples, peeled, thinly sliced and chopped

Instructions

1. With a whisk, mix the dry ingredients (brown rice flour, potato starch, tapioca flour, xanthan gum, baking powder, ground cinnamon, baking soda, ground nutmeg, salt, and sugar) well in a large bowl.
2. In another bowl, give them a whisk to mix the eggs and vegetable oil well. Ensure the kneading blade(s) are correctly attached, and then pour the dough into the baking pan.
3. From Step 1: Pour the flour mixture into the baking pan.
4. Put the baking pan in the home bakery, close the lid, then plug the power cord into the wall. Choose the CAKE class. Set the crust setting for the BB-CEC20, BB-PAC20, and BB-PDC20 to medium and for the BB-HAC10 to regular. Hit START.
5. When the add beeps, open the lid and use a rubber spatula to carefully scrape any flour left on the side of the pan. If the blades are moving, please be careful.
6. Put in the chopped apples and walnuts, put the lid back on, and keep baking. For models BB-HAC10, BB-PAC20, and BB-PDC20, press the START button to get the kneading going again.
7. When it's done, press "Cancel" and take it out of the pan. Let the cake cool before cutting it and serving it.
8. Enjoy!

70. ARTISAN BREAD

Prep Time: 15 Minutes | Cook Time: 30 Minutes

Total Times: 1 Hour 15 Minutes | Serving: 1 Loaf

Ingredients

- gf Jules

Plus:

- 4 1/2 Tbs. sugar (56 grams) or monk fruit sweetener or Swerve or maple sugar
- 1/4 cup of extra virgin olive oil
- 1 1/2 cups of warm water

Toppings (optional):

- flaxseeds or sesame seeds
- coarse sea salt
- egg mixed wiflax seeds or sesame seeds
- coarse sea salt
- oil to brush on top
- egg mixed with 1 Tbs.
- oil to brush on top
- proofing basket (optional)

Instructions

1. Mix oil and water in the wide range bowl of a stand mixer or a separate bowl. Gradually add the gfJules UPDATED Gluten Free Bread. Pour the sugar slowly into the bowl of wet ingredients while mixing with the paddle attachment. Once everything is mixed, add the yeast granules and beat for another 2–3 minutes.
2. Jules Flour and place the dough on it, rolling it gently in the flour to cover all sides. Knead until a smooth ball forms. Sprinkle more gf on a pastry mat or a clean counter.
3. Move to a proofing basket (like the one in the picture), a bowl, or a glass bowl lined with oiled parchment paper.
4. Cover loosely with a warm, damp tea towel or a piece of oiled parchment paper and put in a hot place for 30 minutes to 1 hour to rise.
5. Set the oven temperature to 475°F (static) or 450°F (convection).
6. Move the bread carefully to a baking sheet lined with parchment paper. Flip the bread over so that the bottom of the proofing basket is now the top. Take out the proofing bowl or basket and add more gf.Jules Flour.
7. Wet a large knife with a serrated edge or a dough lame and cut the bread in two or three lines, rocking the knife back and forth to make the cuts wider. You can also use a lame to cut a decorative pattern into the bread. This will give the bread natural places to rise, and it will look even better when it's baked.
8. Bake on the lower rack for 30–35 minutes. Use an instant-read thermometer to ensure it's done before removing it from The oven. The thermometer should have read 205 degrees Fahrenheit.

71. LIGHT MOCK RYE BREAD

Prep Time: 10 Minutes | Cook Time: 30 Minutes

Total Times: 40 Minutes | Serving: 1 Loaf

Ingredients

Wet ingredients:

- 1 1/4 cups of water
- 3 tbsp canola oil
- 3 large eggs, lightly beaten
- 1 1/2 tbsp molasses
- 1 tsp vinegar

Dry ingredients:

- 1/2 cup of non-fat dry milk
- 1 cup of brown rice flour
- 1 tbsp egg replacer (optional)
- 1 (0.25 ounce) package (7g) or 2 1/4 tsp
- 4 tbsp brown sugar, firmly packed
- 1 1/2 tsp salt
- 2 1/4 cups of white rice flour
- 4 tsp caraway seeds
- 1 tbsp xanthan gum

Instructions

1. Confirm that everything is at room temperature. First, using a whisk in a bowl, combine the wet ingredients, and then pour the resulting mixture into a baking dish. Put all the dry ingredients in a separate bowl and whisk them together. Then, place the dry ingredients on top of the wet ingredients in the baking pan.
2. Choose the gluten-free cycle and turn on the machine. After the mixing starts, use a rubber spatula to work any unmixed ingredients into the dough. Stay near the edges and top of the batter to keep the kneading blade from getting in the way.
3. Take the pan out of the machine when the cycle is done.
4. Allow the bread to keep in the pan for approximately 10 minutes, flip it over, and give it a gentle shake to get it out. Before slicing, let it cool, standing up on a rack.

72. NUTS AND SEEDS BREAD

Prep Time: 20 Minutes | Cook Time: 1 Hour 50 Minutes

Total Times: 2 hrs 10 mins | Serving: 1 Loaf

Ingredients

- 1 tbsp millet seeds
- 1 tbsp walnuts
- 350ml water
- 1 tsp cider vinegar
- 4 tsp vegetable oil
- 2 medium eggs
- 1 tbsp linseeds
- 1 tbsp pumpkin seeds
- 1 tbsp sesame seeds
- 1 tsp salt
- 1 tsp honey
- 450g gluten-free bread flour
- 1 1/2 tsp yeast

Instructions

1. Before making the bread, roast the nuts and seeds to bring out their nutty flavor.
2. Now, sprinkle with a little salt and let it cool. (We suggest that you buy a package of each of the seeds and nuts, cook them all together, and then store them in an airtight container when they're cool.
3. They're great for baking or adding flavor and texture to salads. Place water, vinegar, oil, eggs, salt, and sugar in the bread pan.
4. Add the flour, seeds, and yeast, and set your bread maker to make gluten-free bread with a dark crust.

73. SEED BREAD

Prep Time: 30 Minutes | Cook Time: 1 Hour 15 Minutes | Rise Time 1 Hour 15minutes

Total Times: 3 Hour| Serving: 1 Loaf

Ingredients

- 300 ml Cold water (approximately 1 ¼ cups of)
- 30 g Oil (2 tbsp)
- 500 g Gluten-free Brown Bread Mix (4 x 250 ml / 4 cups of)
- 30 ml Pumpkin seeds (2 tbsp)
- 5 ml Salt (1 tsp)
- 30 ml Sugar (2 tbsp)
- 30 ml Poppy seeds (2 tbsp)
- 30 ml Sunflower seeds (2 tbsp)
- 7 g Anchor Instant Yeast (1 packet)

Instructions

1. Take the pan out of the breadmaker.
2. Make sure the paddle is in the place and secure.
3. Put the salt and sugar in the pan along with the cold water.
4. Next, put the pan in the bread machine and add the Gluten-free Brown Bread Mix, pumpkin seeds, sunflower seeds, and poppy seeds.
5. Put the Anchor Instant Yeast in a shallow well you make in the flour.
6. Turn on the machine and press menu 1, which is called "basic setting."
7. Choose a loaf size of 900g/1pound/1.5pound and a medium color.
8. Check the choices and hit the start button.
9. After the cycle is done, take the pan out and then let it cool for nearly 10 minutes. Get out and cool down.
10. Now slice the bread and serve.

74. OATNUT 3-SEED BREAD

Prep Time: 20 Minutes | Cook Time: 3 Hours

Total Times: 5 Hour 20 Minutes | Serving: 1 Loaf

Ingredients

- 1 tsp gluten-free apple cider vinegar
- 1/2 cup of cornstarch
- 1/4 cup of non-fat instant dry milk (or non-fat milk instead of water)
- 1 cup of + 2 tbsp water, at room temperature
- 1/4 cup of neutral-flavored oil
- 2 tbsp honey (or sugar)
- 1 tbsp sesame seeds
- 1 cup of + 2 tbsp potato starch
- 1 tsp poppy seeds
- 1-1/2 cups of certified gluten-free oat flour, plus more for dusting
- 3 large eggs, at room temperature
- 2 tbsp sunflower seeds
- 1 tbsp xanthan gum
- 1 tsp salt
- 2-1/4 tsp instant dry yeast
- 1 tbsp finely chopped hazelnuts (optional)
- 2 tsp gluten-free oats or seeds, for topping (optional)

Instructions

1. First, take the bread pan out of the bread machine and then make sure the paddle is already attached.
2. Put water, dry milk, oil, vinegar, eggs, and honey in a bowl. Mix well.
3. In a separate mixing bowl, nicely mix together the oat flour, potato starch, cornstarch, xanthan gum, sunflower seeds, sesame seeds, poppy seeds, yeast, salt, and hazelnuts (if using).
4. Next, stir the dry mixture into the wet mixture until everything is well mixed.
5. Put the bread pan back in the machine that makes bread. Use the machine's menu button to choose the gluten-free option, then press the "Start" button.
6. Use a clean silicone or rubber spatula to scrape any flour off the sides of the pan during the mixing cycle.
7. When the mixing is done, take out the mixing paddle so that the bottom of the bread doesn't get a big hole. Use the spatula to make a nice smooth top.
8. If you want, you can sprinkle oats or seeds on top of the bread and use wet fingers to gently press them into the dough.
9. When the baking cycle is done, take the hot loaf out of the pan and put it on a clean wire rack. Now, let it cool for at least 2 hours.
10. If the crust is too hard, you can use a clean tea towel to cover it and sides (cover only the top) of the bread while it cools on the rack. This will help make the crust a little bit softer.
11. Once cooled, remove the paddle (if it was left in) using a steak knife. Slice the bread using an electric slicer, electric knife, or serrated knife.
12. It is recommended to slice and freeze any gluten-free bread, although you can store it on the countertop overnight if desired.

75. GOJI BERRIES BREAD

Prep Time: 20 Minutes | Cook Time: 1 Hour 35 Minutes

Total Times: 1 hr 55 mins | Serving: 1 Loaf

Ingredients

For the Dough:

- 450g low-fat curd or quark
- 75g soaked goji berries
- 150g ground almonds
- 75g oat bran
- 45g corn flour
- 7 eggs
- 75g seed and kernel mixture
- 150g ground flaxseeds
- 2 tsp salt
- 21g baking powder

For the Topping:

- 20g seed and kernel mixture

Instructions

1. Start by soaking the goji berries in water for approximately 5 minutes and then drain them well.
2. Remove the bread pan with the kneading blade from the breadmaker.
3. After that, put all of the dough ingredients into the bread pan, except for the topping.
4. NExt, place the bread pan back into the breadmaker, close the lid, select menu 1, and press start.
5. After approximately 10-15 minutes of mixing, press stop and sprinkle the topping evenly over the dough.
6. Select menu 13 on the breadmaker, press start, and then bake the bread for approximately 1 hour and 30 minutes.

76. CHRISTMAS NUT BREAD

Prep Time: 15 Minutes | Cook Time: 1 Hour 45 Minutes

Total Times: 1 Hour 55 Minutes | Serving:

Ingredients

- 50g buckwheat flour
- 1 tsp salt
- ½ cube fresh yeast
- 155g potato starch
- 1 tsp cider vinegar
- 1 tsp carob flour
- 175g KOMEKO rice flour
- 250ml water
- 1 tsp bread spice mix
- 1 tsp maple syrup
- 1 tbsp psyllium husk powder
- 100g mixed nuts
- 2 tbsp rapeseed oil
- 100g yogurt
- 2 tsp baking powder

Instructions

1. First, take the bread pan with the kneading blade out of the bread machine and add all the ingredients from top to bottom.
2. Put the bread pan back into the breadmaker, close the lid, choose program 14 (gluten-free bread), and press the start button.
3. When the programme or timer goes off, take the bread pan out, turn the bread out, and let it cool.

77. CHESTNUT & RICE FLOUR BREAD

Prep Time: 10 Minutes | Cook Time: 1 Hour | Resting Time: 4 Hour

Total Times: 5 Hour 10 Minutes | Serving: 10

Ingredients

- 3 large eggs
- 90g chestnut flour
- 1 tbsp xanthan gum
- 85g potato starch (flour)
- 4 tbsp dried milk powder(or semi-skimmed)
- ½ tbsp caster sugar
- 3 tbsp sunflower oil
- 370ml water
- 1 ½ tsp fine sea salt
- 125g white rice flour
- 150g brown rice flour
- 1 tsp lemon juice
- 23g dried active yeast (1 ½ tbsp + 1 tsp)

Instructions

1. In a bowl, mix together the flours, xanthan gum, sugar, salt, and milk powder.
2. Next, mix the eggs and water with a whisk until the mixture is light and nicely fluffy, then pour it into the breadmaker pan.
3. After that, add the lemon juice and oil to the pan.
4. Spread the flour mixture in an even layer on top of the wet ingredients.
5. On top of the flour mixture, sprinkle the yeast.
6. Set the bread maker to Basic, Large, or Medium Crust and let it cook.
7. When the bread is done making, take it out of the bread machine right away and put it on a clean wire rack to cool.
8. If the dough paddle is stuck, take it off after the loaf has cooled.
9. You can eat it fresh, toast it, or cut it up and freeze it.

78. WALNUT HONEY BREAD

Prep Time: 4 hour | Cook Time: 25 Minutes

Total Times: 4 Hour 25 Minutes | Serving: 2

Ingredients

Wet mixture:

- 3 large eggs
- 3 tbsp vegetable oil
- 3 tbsp honey
- 1 1/4 cups of warm water

Dry mixture:

- 1 cup of tapioca flour
- 1 tbsp xanthan gum
- 1 1/2 cups of garfava bean flour
- 2/3 cup of corn starch
- 1 1/2 tsp salt
- 1/4 cup of walnuts, ground
- 1 (0.25 ounce) package (7g) or 2 1/4 tsp Red Star Active Dry Yeast

Instructions

1. Have all the ingredients at room temperature. Start adding the wet ingredients to the mixing bowl and whisk to combine. Pour the mixture into a baking pan. After that put the dry ingredients in a separate bowl and whisk them together. Next, add the dry ingredients on top of the wet ingredients in the baking pan.
2. Turn on the machine, and choose the gluten-free setting. As soon as the mixer has been turned on, use a rubber spatula to incorporate any unmixed ingredients into the dough, keeping to edges and top of batter to prevent any interference with the kneading blade.
3. When the cycle is done, remove the pan from the machine Now, let the bread stay in the pan for nearly 10 minutes, then flip the pan over and shake it lightly to remove the bread. Cool it upright on a rack before slicing.

79. MOLASSES WALNUT BREAD

Prep Time: 10 Minutes | Cook Time: 2 Hour 30 Minutes

Total Times: 3 Hour | Serving: 1 ounce

Ingredients

- 2 tbsp potato starch
- 1⅓ cups of low-fat milk, room temperature
- 3 tbsp of unsalted butter, room temperature, cut into pieces
- ½ cup of plus 1 tbsp chopped walnuts
- 2 tsp xanthan gum
- 1 tsp gelatin
- 3 tbsp molasses
- 1 large egg, room temperature
- ¾ tsp cider vinegar
- 1½ tsp kosher salt
- 1 cup of garfava flour
- ¾ cup of tapioca flour
- ½ cup of sorghum flour
- ½ cup of plus 1 tbsp cornstarch
- 2¼ tsp yeast, active dry or instant

Instructions

1. First, put all the ingredients into the bread pan with the kneading paddle in the order given.
2. Put the bread pan in the Automatic Bread Maker and lock it in place.
3. To choose the Gluten Free program, press the menu button.
4. To start mixing, rising, and baking, press the Start/Stop button.
5. While the dough is being mixed, use a clean rubber spatula to scrape the sides of the bread pan to make sure all the ingredients are being mixed in.
6. Carefully take the bread pan out of the bread machine when the cycle is done.
7. Set the bread pan on a wire rack to let the bread cools down completely. Now slice it and serve

80. DATE NUT BREAD

Prep Time: 10 Minutes | Cook Time: 2-3 hours | Cooling time: 1 hour

Total Times: 3 hours 10 Minutes-4 hours 10 Minutes | Serving: 16

Ingredients

- 1/2 tsp salt
- 1 tsp vanilla extract
- 1/3 cup of chopped walnuts
- 3/4 cup of chopped dates
- 3 tbsp unsalted butter, 1/2 in. pieces
- 3/4 cup of boiling water
- 2/3 cup of granulated sugar
- 1 1/3 cups of all-purpose flour
- 1 tsp baking soda
- 1 tsp baking powder

Instructions

1. Put the ingredients in the bread pan in the order given. Set the machine to the quick bread/cake setting with a medium crust.
2. After 4 minutes of mixing, use a rubber scraper to stir the sides and bottom of the batter to make sure it is fully mixed.
3. Just before you start baking, stop the machine and take out the paddle if your machine can do this. When the bread is done baking, take it out of the machine and take it on a wire rack to cool. Cool bread slices are best. Cover with plastic wrap to keep food fresh.

81. SUNFLOWER SEED BREAD

Prep Time: 5 Minutes | Cook Time: 3 hours 40 Minutes

Total Times: 3 hours 45 Minutes | Serving: 12-14

Ingredients

- 5 tbsp dark brown soft sugar
- 580 g 4 cups of seeded bread flour
- 2 tsp salt
- 50 g hulled sunflower seeds in the seed tray
- 360 ml 1.5 cups of water
- 3/4 tsp fast-action yeast
- 3 tbsp skimmed milk powder
- 1/2 tsp vitamin C powder
- 3 tbsp sunflower oil

Instructions

1. If your bread machine has a top tray, place the sunflower seeds there. Otherwise, add all the ingredients to the tin and set the machine to the settings you prefer. If not, save the seeds for later, after the first sprout has formed.
2. Go ahead and start the whole wheat loaf.

82. SEEDED BROWN BREAD

Prep Time: 10 Minutes | Cook Time: 2 hours | Cooling time: 1 hour

Total Times: 3 hours Minutes | Serving: 1 loaf

Ingredients

- 2 tsp quick yeast
- 2 tbsp poppy seeds
- 2 tbsp sunflower seeds
- 2 tbsp pumpkin seeds
- FREE Brown Bread Flour 500g
- tepid water 530ml
- 1 tsp vinegar
- 2 tbsp walnut oil
- 4 tbsp sunflower oil
- 1 tsp salt
- 1 tbsp sugar
- 2 egg whites(or FREEE Chickpea Flour & Water) (20g + 40ml)

Instructions

1. Put the egg whites, sugar, salt, oils, vinegar, and water in a bowl and blend until smooth and free of lumps.
2. Put this into the pan for the machine.
3. Mix in the pumpkin, sunflower, and poppy seeds with the flour.
4. The yeast goes on top.
5. Make sure the pan is locked in place, and put the lid on.
6. If there is a gluten-free program, use it. If not, use a basic fast setting.
7. Choose the dark crust if it's an option.
8. Get the machine going.
9. When the bread is done baking, carefully take the pan out of the machine.
10. Remove the mixer paddle from the loaf's bottom by tipping it out of the pan.
11. On a wire rack, let the bread cool.
12. Wait until the bread is cold before cutting it for the best results.

83. FLAXSEED BREAD

Prep Time: 10 Minutes | Cook Time: 2 hours

Total Times: 2 hours 10 Minutes | Serving: 16

Ingredients

- 2 1/2 tsp xanthan gum
- 1 1/2 tsp salt
- 1/4 cup of brown rice flour
- 3 large eggs
- 1/2 cup of milk powder
- 1 cup of tapioca flour
- 3 Tbsp sugar
- 1 2/3 cup of water
- 1/2 cup of ground flaxseed flour
- 3 Tbsp oil
- 2 1/4 tsp yeast
- 1 tsp vinegar
- 1 1/2 cup of corn flour

Instructions

1. In a bread pan, put eggs, water, milk powder, sugar, oil, and vinegar.
2. Flour, xanthan gum, and salt are mixed together well in a bowl with a whisk. Add to the bread pan.
3. Make a well on top and pour the yeast into it.
4. Choose a song with only one rise cycle.

84. LINSEED BROWN BREAD

Prep Time: 20 Minutes | Cook Time: 2-3 hours

Total Times: 2-3 hours 20 Minutes | Serving: 1 loaf

Ingredients

- 3tbsp dry milk powder
- 50g quinoa flour
- 1½tsp salt
- 2tsp light brown sugar
- 225g brown rice flour
- 1tsp lemon juice
- 50g buckwheat flour
- 1tbsp active dried yeast
- 1 tsp xantham gum
- 1tbsp linseed
- 1tbsp black treacle
- 3tbsp sunflower oil
- 350ml water
- 1 large egg
- 1tbsp gluten-free baking powder

Instructions

1. To make a smooth paste, combine the egg, milk powder, and water in a bowl. Whisk until combined. Pour into the breadmaker's pan.
2. Put the lemon juice, sugar, syrup, and oil on. Then put the flour, gum, linseed, and salt on top. Finally, sprinkle the yeast over everything.
3. Start your bread machine on the basic setting for a medium (up to 700g) loaf with a dark crust if you can. Let the bread machine do what it's best at.
4. When the loaf is done, let it cool down on a rack for at least ten minutes and then eat it. Gluten-free brown bread with linseed should be good for at least four days.

85. BROWN RICE MILLET BREAD

Prep Time: 15 Minutes | Cook Time: 1-2 hour | Additional time: 2-3 hours

Total Times: 3-5 hours 15 Minutes | Serving: 8-12

Ingredients

- Tapioca Starch - 163g (1 ¼ cup)
- Honey (room temperature) - 2 tbsp
- Liquids (room temperature) - 2 Large Eggs + Milk (300g/300ml, 1 ¼ cup)
- Instant Dry Yeast - 1 tsp (3g)
- Millet Flour - 37g (¼ cup)
- Xanthan Gum - 1 ½ tsp (4.5g)
- Brown Rice Flour - 162g (1 ⅓ cup)
- Cider Vinegar - 1 ½ tsp
- Olive Oil - 2 ½ tbsp
- Salt - 1 tsp

Instructions

1. First, put Tapioca Starch into the bread machine so that it can dissolve completely in water. Combine the Eggs and Milk in a measuring cup. First, put the eggs in the measuring cup. Then, add enough milk to get to the right weight or volume (300g/300ml, 1 14 cups).
2. Pour the mixture of the egg and milk into the bread machine.
3. Add Olive Oil, Honey, Cider Vinegar, Salt, Brown Rice Flour, Millet Flour, Xanthan Gum, and then Instant Dry Yeast.
4. Make a hole in the flour mixture to hold the yeast, and make sure it doesn't touch the liquids.
5. Stop the lid of the bread machine and choose the bread setting and crust color you want.
6. Start the bread machine and let it knead, rise, and bake according to the machine's instructions for the setting you chose.
7. After baking, carefully remove the bread from the bread machine and cool it down on a wire rack before slicing and serving.

86. PSYLLIUM HUSK BREAD

Prep Time: 15 Minutes | Cook Time: 2 hours 15 Minutes

Total Times: 2 hours 30 Minutes | Serving: 1 loaf

Ingredients

- 2 eggs at room temperature and beaten
- ¼ cup of (40g) unsalted butter, room temperature and cut into small cubes
- 1 tsp (5g) baking powder
- 1 cup of (240g) warm water
- 3 tbsp (18g) psyllium husk
- 2 tsp (6g) xanthan gum
- ½ cup of + ½ tbsp (75g) brown rice flour
- 1 ¼ cup of (155g) millet flour
- 1 tsp (7g) salt
- 2 tsp (8g) active dry yeast
- 1 ¼ cup of + 2 tbsp (160g) tapioca starch
- 2 tbsp (28g) sugar

Instructions

1. Mix the water, active dry yeast, and sugar in a small bowl. Leave it alone for 10 minutes to get the yeast to work. If the solution doesn't have a little bit of foam, the yeast is dead, and you'll need to get some more.
2. Mix the tapioca starch, millet flour, brown rice flour, salt, psyllium husk, baking powder, and xanthan gum in a bowl that's about the size of a salad bowl. Combine everything together, then set the bowl aside.
3. After the yeast has grown, add the egg and butter that have been beaten.
4. First, put the wet ingredients into the bread machine, then the dry ones.
5. Choose the gluten-free setting on the bread maker (or similar appliance), close the lid, and press the start button.
6. Remove the paddle (optional) if you are warned, then take a spatula to spread the dough out evenly in the pan.
7. After baking, take the loaf out of the oven and take it on a cooling rack to cool completely.
8. Enjoy!

87. FRENCH BREAD

Prep Time: 10 Minutes | Total Times: 180 Minutes

Serving: 8-12 slices

Ingredients

- 7g dry yeast or 12 g fresh yeast
- 5g salt
- 350g Mix Bread
- 20g butter
- 350ml water
- 20g honey

Instructions

1. Gather the ingredients for gluten-free bread.
2. Next, add the ingredients to the bread machine in the specified order.
3. Close the lid of the bread machine.
4. Set the desired program on the bread machine.
5. Press the "Start" button.
6. Let the bread machine complete the cycle.
7. Remove the baked bread from the machine.
8. After that allow the bread to cool for a few minutes.
9. Slice the bread generously.
10. Spread your favorite topping on each slice.
11. Enjoy your homemade gluten-free bread!

88. VEGAN BREAD

Prep Time: 15 Minutes | Cook Time: 70 Minutes

Total Times: 1 Hour 25 Minutes | Serving: 1 Loaf or 12 slices

Ingredients

- 1/2 cup of potato starch (70g)
- 1/2 cup of tapioca flour* (60g)
- 1 tbsp of organic coconut palm sugar or maple syrup (10g)
- 1 cup of buckwheat flour (120-130g)
- 1-1/4 cup of homemade hemp milk (300g)
- 1/2 tbsp fine grey sea salt (8g)
- 1/2 cup of white rice flour (70g)
- 1/2 cup of brown rice flour (70g)
- 2 tsp active yeast (10g)
- 1/2 cup of seed or nut flour(50-60g)
- 2 tbsp whole psyllium husk (14g)
- 1 cup of warm water (240g)

Instructions

1. Before you start the preparation, you can watch the bread machine loaf video tutorial. And before you start, make sure to measure and sift all the dry ingredients. This step is essential if you don't want starch or flour lumps in your loaf.
2. Mix the yeast, psyllium husk, and warm water together in a large bowl. You can wait 5 minutes or add the rest of the dry ingredients right away.
3. Again, to ensure that all of your ingredients are thoroughly sifted, place a sieve over the top of your mixing bowl and then add the dry ingredients one at a time.
4. Take off the sieve and mix the ingredients gently. Start by adding 1 cup of hemp milk and mixing until all of the dry and wet ingredients are well combined.
5. We don't want any dry bits of flour to be left at the bottom. If your mix is still a little dry, add the last 1/4 cup of hemp milk. Finish mixing until everything is well-mixed.
6. Next, let the dough rise right in the bowl or you can move the mixture to the pan of the bread machine.
7. After that make sure to scrape down the sides of the bowl, cover it, and then let the dough rise in a warmer place for around 2 hours or until it has grown more than an inch tall or even doubled in size.
8. When you're ready to bake, carefully move the dough to the bread machine pan, if it's not already there, and bake it for at least 1 hour and 10 minutes. Your bread machine will be set to "bake only."
9. Take the bread out of the pan when it's done and set it on a cooling rack to cool for few hours, or until it's cold all the way through. Eat it by slicing it up.

89. ITALIAN HERB BREAD

Prep Time: 2 Hours 25 Minutes | Cook Time: Minutes

Total Times: 2 Hours 25 Minutes | Serving: 1 Loaf or 12 slices

Ingredients

- 3 Tbsp Honey
- 1 Tbsp Xanthan Gum
- 1 1/2 Cup of Milk
- 3 Tbsp Olive Oil
- 3 Large Eggs, beaten
- 1 Tbsp Apple Cider Vinegar
- 1 1/2 Tsp Salt
- 1 1/2 Cup of Brown Rice Flour
- 2 1/3 Cups of Potato Starch
- 3 Tsp Italian Seasoning (oregano, basil, thyme, garlic powder, onion powder)
- 1 Tbsp Rapid Raise Active Dry Yeast

Instructions

1. Add the ingredients to the loaf pan of the Zojirishi bread machine in the order given.
2. Set the machine to the Gluten-Free setting and let it make the loaf of bread for you. (Always follow the instructions or guide that came with the bread maker.)
3. Now, let the bread cool in the pan before taking it out and cutting it.
4. Enjoy the tasty food!

90. RICE FLOUR & BUCKWHEAT BREAD

Prep Time: 20 Minutes | Cook Time: Minutes

Total Times: 5 Hours | Serving: 1 Loaf or 12 slices

Ingredients

- 25g linseed
- 335g KOMEKO rice flour
- 25g KOMEKO rice flour
- 10g salt
- 1¼ tsp dry yeast
- 25g buckwheat seeds
- 100g hot water
- 25g oil
- 25g syrup
- 100g buckwheat flour
- bread spice
- 300g water

Instructions

1. First, roast 25 grams of buckwheat seeds, then add 100 grams of hot water (it should hiss), and mix in 25 grams of linseed. Give it 3 hours to soak.
2. Next, take the bread pan with the kneading blade out of the breadmaker and then add all of the dry ingredients from the given list. The last step is to add the liquids to the seeds that have been soaking.
3. Put the bread pan back into the breadmaker, close the lid, choose menu list, and press the start button.
4. Around 50 minutes before the end of the baking time, add water to the bread to make it more moist. Then, sprinkle it with linseed and lightly press it with the back of your hand.
5. When the bread is done, press the "Stop" button and then unplug the machine.
6. Using dry oven gloves, remove the bread immediately and put it on a clean wire rack so that it can cool down.

91. SESAME BREAD

Prep Time: 10 Minutes | Cook Time: Minutes

Total Times: 2 Hours | Serving: 1 Loaf or 8-12 slices

Ingredients

- 1¼ tsp dry yeast
- 300g water
- 10g salt
- 50g buckwheat flour
- 375g KOMEKO rice flour
- 40g treacle
- 75g sesame
- 10g cider vinegar

Topping:

- sesame

Instructions

1. At first, roast 75g of sesame, then let it cool.
2. Now, take the bread pan with the kneading blade out of the breadmaker and then add all of the dry ingredients, including the sesame seeds, in the order given. The last step is to add the liquids.
3. Put the bread pan back into the breadmaker, close the lid, choose menu list, and press the start button.
4. Nearly 50 minutes before the end of the baking time, add water to the bread to make it more moist. Then sprinkle it with sesame seeds and press it gently with your hand.
5. When the bread is done, press the "Stop" button and then unplug the machine.
6. Using dry oven gloves, remove the bread from the oven immediately and set it on a wire rack to cool.

92. PUMPKIN BREAD

Prep Time: 10 Minutes | Cook Time: Minutes

Total Times: 2 Hours | Serving: 1 Loaf or 8-12 slices

Ingredients

- 1 ¼ tsp dry yeast
- 250g KOMEKO rice flour
- 50g pumpkin seeds
- 100g potato starch
- 200g pumpkin
- 110g buckwheat flour
- ginger / nutmeg
- 100g water
- 15g salt

Topping:

- pumpkin seeds

Instructions

1. Steam the pumpkin with 100g of water, then use a fork to make a puree or crush it. Add enough water so that the total weight is about 375g.
2. Next, take the bread pan with the kneading blade out of the breadmaker and then add all of the dry ingredients in the listed order. Last, put in the pumpkin puree.=
3. Put the bread pan back into the breadmaker, close the lid, choose menu list, and press the start button.
4. Almost 50 minutes before the end of the baking time, add water to the bread to make it more moist. Then sprinkle on the chopped pumpkin seeds and lightly press them with the back of your hand.
5. When the bread is done, press the "Stop" button and then unplug the machine.
6. Using dry oven gloves, remove the bread from the oven immediately and set it on a wire rack to cool.

93. VEGAN CINNAMON RAISIN BREAD

Prep Time: 10 Minutes | Cook Time: Minutes

Total Times: 3 Hours | Serving: 1 Loaf or 8-12 slices

Ingredients

- 1 1/2 tsp salt
- 3 tbsp vegetable oil
- 4 cups of all purpose flour
- 1/3 cup of plant milk
- 1/4 cup of granulated sugar
- 1 1/3 cup of water
- 1 1/4 cup of raisins
- 1 1/2 tsp ground cinnamon
- 2 tsp bread machine yeast

Instructions

1. Start adding all of the ingredients EXCEPT raisins into the bread machine, in the order we have suggested in your bread machines manual.
2. Choosing the "Sweet" cycle.
3. When the machine beeps the "add ingredient" signal, put the raisins in.

94. GARLIC BREAD

Prep Time: 15 Minutes | Cook Time: Minutes

Total Times: 2-3 Hours | Serving: 1 Loaf or 8-12 slices

Ingredients

Wet Ingredients:

- 3/4 cup of dairy free milk
- 1 + 1/2 Tbsp. maple syrup
- 6 – 7 cloves of garlic, minced
- 2 tbsp of flax meal plus 6 tbsp warm water, mix and let stand for 5 min
- 1 + 1/2 tsp. apple cider vinegar
- 2 Tbsp. vegan butter (earth balance)
- roughly 1/8 cups of parsley, loosely chopped

Dry Ingredients:

- 1 + 2/3 cups of brown rice flour
- 1 Tbsp. garlic powder
- 1 Tbsp. onion powder
- 1/4 cup of corn starch
- 2 Tbsp. potato starch
- 1 + 1/2 tsp. xanthan gum
- 1/2 tsp. salt

Yeast:

- 1 tsp. active dry yeast

Instructions

1. Mix the flax eggs together and let them sit for 5 minutes.
2. In the meantime, mix the dry ingredients (brown rice flour, corn starch, potato starch, xanthan gum, onion/garlic powders, and salt) in a separate bowl.
3. Pour wet ingredients like milk, flax eggs, apple cider vinegar, vegan butter, maple syrup, minced garlic, and parsley into the bread machine.
4. Put the dry mixture on top of the wet mixture in the bread machine, completely covering the liquid
5. Next, create a small well in the middle of the dry mixture and put the yeast in it, making sure it doesn't touch any liquid.
6. Cook on the white bread/light crust setting, or follow the exact instructions that came with your bread machine.
7. When the bread is done, remove it immediately from the bread machine because it can burn if left in there for too long. Put on cooling rack to cool completely (away from the cat) before putting in an airtight container. Will last about 4 days or longer if kept in the refrigerator.
8. Serve lightly toasted, maybe with a tomato-based or Alfredo pasta, or serve lightly toasted with avocado slices.

95. BANANA BREAD WITH PUMPKIN

Prep Time: 7 Minutes | Cook Time: Minutes

Total Times: 1 Hour 7 Minutes | Serving: 1 Loaf or 8-12 slices

Ingredients

- 50g tapioca starch
- 1/2 organic orange
- 25g peanut oil
- 230g pumpkin
- 1 tsp of ground cinnamon
- 1scant /2 tsp of ground ginger
- 8g ground linseed
- 35g dark muscovado sugar
- 30g rolled oats

- a pinch of salt
- 1 banana
- 45g almond flour
- 3g bicarbonate of soda
- 1 tbsp of orange juice
- 85g rice syrup
- 6g cream of tartar
- 70g wholegrain sorghum flour

Instructions

1. First preheat the oven to 180°C.
2. Now, use baking paper to line the tin.
3. To make medium oatmeal, grind the rolled oats. You can also grind the almonds and linseed to obtain flour.
4. Add the flours, baking soda, cream of tartar, sugar, salt, and spices in a powerful food processor. Then start and mix, 40 to 50 seconds is enough.
5. Add all of the wet ingredients—syrup, oil, orange juice, banana pieces, and finally pumpkin—and mix well until the mixture is thick and smooth. (For better results, mix the wet and dry ingredients separately and then mix them together. Important: Don't blend for too long. 60–90 seconds is enough to mix all the ingredients and get rid of any pumpkin or banana lumps. If it's not enough, mash it with a fork and scrape the sides with a spatula.
6. Next, pour the mixture into the cake tin and use the spatula to make it even.
7. Brush a small amount of syrup and plant milk (optional) over the top. Put a handful of pumpkin seeds on top, lightly press them into the mixture so they don't stick out, and then brush the top again.
8. Bake for at least 55 to 60 minutes at 180°C. Before bringing it out of the oven, test it with a clean skewer to make sure it comes out clean and moist, with no mixture stuck to it. Let the bread cool in the tin before taking it out.

96. BROWN RICE VEGAN BREAD

Prep Time: 15 Minutes | Cook Time: Minutes

Total Times: 2 hours and 30 minutes | Serving: 1 Loaf or 8-12 slices

Ingredients

- 254g (1 ¾ cup of) Potato Starch
- 300g (300ml, 1 ¼ cup of) Water (room temperature)
- 2 ½ tbsp Olive Oil (can be substituted with other vegetable oils)
- 2 tbsp Maple Syrup (room temperature)
- 1 tsp Salt
- 125g (1 cup of) Brown Rice Flour
- 1 ½ tsp Xanthan Gum
- 1 tsp Instant Dry Yeast (no contact with liquids)

Instructions

1. Add potato starch to the bread machine to dissolve in water. Pour room temperature water into the bread machine.
2. Add olive oil to the bread machine. Add maple syrup to the bread machine. Sprinkle salt into the bread machine.
3. Add brown rice flour to the bread machine.
4. Sprinkle xanthan gum evenly over the flour mixture and mix well.
5. Create a small indentation on top of the flour mixture for the yeast.
6. Carefully add the instant dry yeast to the indentation without touching any liquids.
7. Place the bread machine pan into the machine and close the lid. Set the bread machine menu to "Gluten Free." Choose the desired crust setting, preferably "Medium."
8. Select the appropriate loaf size: 2.0 POUND, 1.5 POUND, or 1.0 POUND. Set the cooking time to 2 hours and 10 minutes (2:10). Start the bread machine to begin the baking process.
9. Once the machine beeps, carefully remove the bread pan. Now, let the bread cool downs nicely in the pan for several minutes before transferring it to a cooling rack.
10. After that let the bread cool completely on the rack before slicing it into pieces and serving it.

97. QUINOA CHICKPEA VEGAN BREAD

Prep Time: 15 Minutes | Cook Time: Minutes

Total Times: 3 hours and 30 minutes | Serving: 1 Loaf or 8-12 slices

Ingredients

- 144g (1 ⅛ cup of) Cornstarch
- 44g (⅓ cup of) Quinoa Flour
- 2 ½ tbsp Olive Oil (can be substituted with other vegetable oils)
- 2 tbsp Maple Syrup (room temperature)
- 50g (⅜ cup of) Chickpea Flour
- 4.5g (1 ½ tsp) Xanthan Gum
- 140g (⅞ cup of) White Rice Flour
- 1 tsp Instant Dry Yeast (no contact with liquids)
- 320g (320ml, 1 ⅓ cup of) Water (room temperature)
- 1 tsp Salt

Instructions

1. Add the Cornstarch (144g) to the bread machine first to allow the starch to fully dissolve in water.
2. Pour the Water (320g) at room temperature into the bread machine.
3. Add the Olive Oil (2 ½ tbsp) to the bread machine. It can be substituted with other vegetable oils.
4. Add the Maple Syrup (2 tbsp) at room temperature to the bread machine.
5. Sprinkle the Salt (1 tsp) into the bread machine.
6. Add the Quinoa Flour (44g) to the bread machine.
7. Add the Chickpea Flour (50g) to the bread machine.
8. Add the White Rice Flour (140g) to the bread machine.
9. Sprinkle the Xanthan Gum (4.5g) evenly over the flour mixture. Mix well with all the flour ingredients.
10. Create a small indentation on top of the flour mixture to hold the Instant Dry Yeast.
11. Carefully add the Instant Dry Yeast (1 tsp) to the indentation, then making sure it does not get contact with any liquids.
12. Place the bread machine pan into the bread machine and close the lid.
13. Set the bread machine menu to the appropriate setting for gluten-free bread.
14. Choose the desired crust setting, such as medium.
15. Select the appropriate loaf size based on the options available.
16. Start the bread machine to begin the baking process according to the recommended cooking time for gluten-free bread.
17. Once the bread machine beeps to indicate that the bread is done, carefully remove the bread pan.

18. After that allow the bread to cool in the pan for a several minutes before moving it to a cooling rack.
19. Now, let the bread cool completely on the rack before slicing and serving.

98. BROWN RICE BREAD

Prep Time: 15 Minutes | Cook Time: Minutes

Total Times: 2-3 Hours | Serving: 1 Loaf or 8-12 slices

Ingredients

- 1/4 cup of (35g) potato starch
- 150g or 3 large eggs, beaten
- 2 Tbsp. (40g) honey
- 1 Tbsp. (14mL) apple cider vinegar
- 1 tsp. (5.6g) salt
- 1/8 cup of (27g) vegetable oil
- 3-1/4 cups of (481g) brown rice flour
- 1-1/2 cups of (360mL) milk
- 1/2 cup of (70g) cornstarch
- 1 Tbsp. (8g) xanthan gum
- 1 Tbsp. (8.5g) active dry yeast

Instructions

1. With a whisk, mix the brown rice flour, corn starch, potato starch, and xanthan gum well in a large bowl.
2. Make sure the kneading blade(s) are attached properly and add the liquid ingredients (milk, beaten eggs, apple cider vinegar, vegetable oil, and honey).
3. Add the mixture of flour and salt from step 1 to the baking pan. With a large spoon, make a small hole in the flour and then put the yeast there. Make sure the yeast doesn't touch any liquid.
4. Put the baking pan in the Home Bakery, close the lid, and then plug the power cord into an outlet.
5. Choose the setting GLUTEN FREE. Set the crust control to how dark you want the crust to be, then press START.
6. When the machine beeps, open the lid and use a clean rubber spatula to push any flour off the sides of the baking pan. Put the lid on. Press and hold the START/RESET or CANCEL button when the baking is done to turn off the Home Bakery. Using oven mitts, remove the loaf from the baking pan and gently shake it out. Let the bread cool, then serve.

99. CASSAVA CENTURY BREAD

Prep Time: 20 Minutes | Cook Time: 3 Hour 30 Minutes

Total Times: 3 Hour 50 Minutes | Serving: 1 Loaf or 8-12 slices

Ingredients

Wet Ingredients:

- 1 1/2 cups of warm almond or coconut milk (very warm to the wrist)
- 1 tsp apple cider vinegar
- 3 eggs
- 1 Tbsp honey, molasses, or maple syrup
- 1/2 cup of melted ghee, butter, or coconut oil

Dry Ingredients:

- 1/2 cup of potato starch
- 2 tsp rapid rise bread machine yeast
- 1/4 cup of flax seed meal
- 1/1/2 tsp psyllium husk or 1 tsp of psyllium powder
- 1/2 cup of arrowroot or tapioca starch
- 1/4 cup of mixed seeds (optional)
- 1-2 tsp Himalayan salt (I use 2)
- 1 1/2 cup of cassava flour

Instructions

Wet Ingredients:

1. Make sure ingredients you're using is at room temperature before you start and that the almond or coconut milk is very warm. After that whisk the wet ingredients together in a bowl until they are well mixed. Set this aside while you mix the dry ingredients next.

Dry Ingredients:

1. Set aside the Active Dry Yeast.
2. Mix the cassava flour, starches, and salt in a medium bowl using a sifter.
3. Mix in the flax seed meal and the seeds with a whisk to make sure they are well mixed.lacing in the Bread Machine
4. Put the warm Wet Ingredients into the pan of the bread machine.
5. Pour the Dry Ingredients, which have been sifted and whisked, over the Wet Ingredients.
6. Use your finger to make a hole and sprinkle the Active Dry Yeast in it.
7. If your machine has a setting for "Gluten-Free," use that setting. If not have a gluten free setting, use the setting #1 (about 3 hours 25 minutes), a large loaf, and top brown.

100. COCONT FLOUR BREAD

Prep Time: 15 Minutes | Cook Time: Minutes

Total Times: 2 to 3 hours | Serving: 1 Loaf or 8-12 slices

Ingredients

- 1 tbsp of honey
- ½ cup of grated coconut plus a ¼ cup of in reserve for topping
- ¾ cup of coconut flour
- 6 eggs at room temperature
- ½ cup of coconut oil or vegetable oil
- ½ tsp of salt
- 1 tbsp of baking powder
- 2 tbsp of arrowroot flour (optional)

Instructions

1. At first add the ingredients to the bread pan in the order shown in the "ingredients" section and choose the cake or batter bread course for a 1-pound loaf with a medium crust. When the kneading cycle is done, sprinkle the last 1/4 cup of coconut flakes on top before starting the baking cycle. When the bread is done, then take the pan out of the machine and let it sit for 10 minutes. After that, remove the bread out of the pan and let it sit for additional 5 minutes on a clean wire rack or cutting board. Slice, then serve.

101. BROWN RICE AND CRANBERRY BREAD

Prep Time: 15 Minutes | Cook Time: Minutes

Total Times: 2 to 3 hours | Serving: 1 Loaf or 8-12 slices

Ingredients

Wet ingredients:

- 1 1/2 cups of water
- 1 tsp cider vinegar
- 3 tsp canola oil
- 3 large eggs, slightly beaten

Dry ingredients:

- 3 cups of brown rice flour
- 1/4 cup of soy flour
- 3 tbsp sugar
- 1 tbsp egg replacer (optional)
- 1/2 cup of dry milk
- 2/3 cup of dried cranberries
- 1 tbsp xantham gum
- 1 1/2 tsp table salt
- 1 (0.25 ounce) package (7g) or 2 1/4 tsp Red Star Active Dry Yeast

Instructions

1. First, make sure that everything is at room temperature. Next, mix the wet ingredients in a bowl with a whisk, after that pour the mixture into a baking pan. Put the dry ingredients in a separate mixing bowl and whisk them together.
2. Following that put the dry ingredients on top of the wet ingredients in the baking pan.
3. Choose the gluten-free cycle and turn on the machine. After the mixing starts, use a rubber spatula to work any unmixed ingredients into the dough. Stay near the edges and top of the batter to keep the kneading blade from getting in the way.
4. Take the pan out of the machine when the cycle is done. Now, let the bread stay in the pan for around 10 minutes, then turn the pan over and give it a light shake to get the bread out. Before slicing, let it cool standing up on a rack.

102. MILLET CHIA BREAD

Prep Time: 15 Minutes | Cook Time: 2 Hour 15 Minutes

Total Times: 2 to 3 hours | Serving: 1 Loaf or 8-12 slices

Ingredients

Dry Ingredients:

- 1 cup of brown rice flour (127g)
- 1/2 cup of cornstarch (70g)
- 1 cup of tapioca flour/starch (120g)
- 1 cup of millet flour (136g)
- 2 tbsp chia seeds
- 1 tbsp flax seed meal
- 1-1/2 tbsp evaporated cane juice (or sugar)
- 1-1/2 tsp guar gum
- 1-1/2 tsp xanthan gum
- 1-1/2 tsp pea protein
- 1-1/2 tsp apple fiber/pectin
- 1 tsp salt
- 2-1/2 tsp instant dry yeast

Wet Ingredients:

- 1-1/2 cups of water
- 1/4 cup of neutral-flavored oil
- 1 tsp unsulphured molasses
- 1/2 cup of egg whites
- 1 tsp apple cider vinegar

Instructions

1. First, put all the dry ingredients into the bread maker's bowl.
2. In a different mixing bowl, mix all the dry ingredients together with a whisk. On top of the wet mixture, put the dry mixture.
3. Set your bread machine to make gluten-free bread and bake it as directed. I set the timer on my Breadman machine for 20 minutes to help me stir the dough and get the dry flour off the bowl's sides and bottom.
4. Then I set another timer for 11 minutes to take out the paddle. From heating the bowl to baking, stirring, rising, and baking, the whole process takes 3 hours.
5. Now, take the bread out of the bowl and then let it cool for minimum of an hour before cutting it.
6. Use a serrated knife, an electric slicer, or an electric knife to cut up the food.
7. Freeze the remaining slices and when needed warm them in the microwave to return their freshness.

103. BUCKWHEAT BREAD

Prep Time: 10 Minutes | Cook Time: 1 Hour 10 Minutes

Total Times: 1 Hours 20 Minuite | Serving: 1 Loaf or 8-12 slices

Ingredients

- 3 eggs
- 3 tbsp. Softened butter
- 1 ½ cups of milk (110° F./43° C.)
- 1 tsp. Soy lecithin
- 1 tbsp. xanthan gum
- 1 tsp. sea salt
- 1 ½ cups of brown rice flour
- ½ cup of potato starch (omit if pure buckwheat bread)
- ½ cup of buckwheat flour (or 3 cups of for pure buckwheat bread)
- ½ cup of tapioca flour (omit if pure buckwheat bread)
- 1 tbsp. Bread machine yeast or active dry yeast

Instructions

1. Start by adding the ingredients to the bread machine in the order given. For a 1.5-pound loaf with a medium crust, you should use the gluten-free setting or the basic white bread setting.
2. When the bread is done, let it sit for 10 minutes. Slice, then serve.

104. BUTTERMILK BREAD

Prep Time: 10 Minutes | Cook Time: 2 Hour 20 Minutes

Total Times: 2-3 Hours | Serving: 1 Loaf or 8-12 slices

Ingredients

Wet ingredients:

- 1 cup of buttermilk
- 3 large eggs (lightly beaten)
- 1/4 cup of plus 1 tbsp water
- 1/4 cup of canola oil (may substitute melted butter, cooled to room temperature)

Dry ingredients:

- 1/2 cup of tapioca flour
- 3 1/2 tsp xanthan gum
- 1/4 cup of granulated sugar
- 2 cups of brown rice flour
- 1/2 cup of potato starch
- 1 1/2 tsp salt
- 1 tbsp egg replacer (optional)
- 1 (0.25 ounce) package (7g) or 2 1/4 tsp Red Star Active Dry Yeast

Instructions

1. Start by making sure that everything is at room temperature. Next, mix the wet ingredients in a bowl with a whisk nicely and then pour the mixture into a baking pan. After that put the dry ingredients in a separate bowl and whisk them together. Then, in the baking pan, put the dry ingredients on top of the wet ingredients.
2. Choose the gluten-free cycle and turn on the machine. After the mixing starts, use a rubber spatula to work any unmixed ingredients into the dough. Make sure to stay away from the kneading blade by keeping to the edges and top of the batter while using the spatula.
3. Take the pan out of the machine when the cycle is done. Now, let the bread stay in the pan for about 10 minutes, then flip the pan over and give it a light shake to get the bread out. Before slicing, let it cools down on a rack.

105. BROWN AND WHITE BREAD

Prep Time: 15 Minutes | Cook Time: 1 Hour 45 Minutes

Total Times: 2 Hours | Serving: 1 Loaf or 8-12 slices

Ingredients

Wet ingredients:

- 1/4 cup of vegetable oil
- 3 large eggs
- 1 tsp cider vinegar
- 1 2/3 cups of water

Dry ingredients:

- 1 cup of brown rice flour
- 2 1/2 tsp xanthan gum
- 2 1/4 cups of white rice flour
- 1/2 cup of dry milk powder
- 1 1/2 tsp salt
- 3 tbsp granulated sugar
- 1 (0.25 ounce) package (7g) or 2 1/4 tsp Red Star Active Dry Yeast

Instructions

1. Ensure that everything is at room temperature. Mix all of the wet ingredients, then pour the mixture into a baking pan. Separately, whisk together the dry ingredients in a separate bowl. Then, in the baking pan, put the dry ingredients on top of the wet ingredients.
2. Choose the gluten-free cycle and turn on the machine. After the mixing starts, use a rubber spatula to work any unmixed ingredients into the dough. Stay near the edges and top of the batter to keep the kneading blade from getting in the way.
3. Take the pan out of the machine when the cycle is done. After letting the bread sit in the pan for approximately 10 minutes, turn it over and gently shake it to remove the bread. Before slicing, let it cool, standing up on a rack.

106. SALT FREE WHITE RICE BREAD

Prep Time: 15 Minutes | Cook Time: Minutes

Total Times: 3 to 4 hours | Serving: 1 Loaf or 8-12 slices

Ingredients

- 330g (330ml, 1 ⅜ cup of) Liquids (room temperature)
- 160g (1 ¼ cup of) Cornstarch
- 2 ½ tbsp Olive Oil (can be substituted with other vegetable oils)
- 2 tbsp Honey (room temperature)
- 1 ½ tsp Cider Vinegar
- 2 Large Eggs + Milk (put eggs in the measuring cup of first, then add milk to the required weight or volume)
- 100g (⅝ cup of) White Rice Flour
- 1 tsp Salt
- 86g (⅝ cup of) Gluten-Free Flour (should not contain pre-added xanthan gum)
- 1 ½ tsp Xanthan Gum (4.5g)
- 1 tsp Instant Dry Yeast (no contact with liquids)

Instructions

1. Add the Cornstarch (160g) to the bread machine first to allow the starch to fully dissolve in milk.
2. Measure the Liquids (330g) at room temperature (Egg(s) + Milk). Put the egg(s) in the measuring cup of first, and then add milk to reach the required weight or volume.
3. Add the Olive Oil (2 ½ tbsp) to the bread machine. It can be substituted with other vegetable oils.
4. Add the Honey (2 tbsp) at room temperature to the bread machine.
5. Add the Cider Vinegar (1 ½ tsp) to the bread machine.
6. Sprinkle the Salt (1 tsp) into the bread machine.
7. Add the Gluten-Free Flour (86g) to the bread machine. Make sure it does not contain pre-added xanthan gum.

8. Add the White Rice Flour (100g) to the bread machine.
9. Sprinkle the Xanthan Gum (1 ½ tsp) evenly over the flour mixture. Mix well with all the flour ingredients.
10. Create a small indentation on top of the flour mixture to hold the Instant Dry Yeast.
11. Carefully add the Instant Dry Yeast (1 tsp) to the indentation,then making sure it does not come into contact with any liquids.
12. Place the bread machine pan into the bread machine and close the lid.
13. Set the bread machine menu to the appropriate setting for gluten-free bread.
14. Start the bread machine to begin the baking process according to the recommended cooking time for gluten-free bread.
15. Once the bread machine beeps to indicate that the bread is done, carefully remove the bread pan.
16. Now, allow the bread to cool in the pan for a several minutes before transferring it to a cooling rack.
17. Let the bread cool completely on a clean rack before slicing and serving.

107. HAMBURGER BUNS

Prep Time: 15 Minutes | Cook Time: 2-3 Minutes

Total Times: 2-3 Minutes | Serving: 8 buns

Ingredients

- 3 large eggs (slightly beaten)
- 3 tbsp vegetable oil
- 1 (0.25 ounce) package of (7g) or 2 1/4 tsp of Red Star Active Dry Yeast
- 1 1/2 tsp salt
- 1 1/4 cup of water
- 1/3 cup of rice flour
- 3 tbsp honey
- 2/3 cup of tapioca flour
- 1 tbsp xanthan gum
- 1 1/2 cup of garfava bean (or garbanzo bean flour)
- 1/2 cup of cornstarch (or arrowroot flour)

Instructions

1. Check sure that everything is at room temperature. Take the wet ingredients in a bowl with a whisk, then put the mixture into a baking pan. Take all the dry ingredients in a separate bowl and whisk them together. Then, Take the dry ingredients on top of the wet ingredients in the baking pan.
2. Choose the gluten-free cycle and turn on the machine. After the mixing starts, use a rubber spatula to work any unmixed ingredients into the dough. Stay near the edges and top of the batter to keep the kneading blade from getting in the way.
3. Take the pan out of the machine when the cycle is done, then the bread stays in the pan for around ten minutes, then flip the pan over and provide it a gentle shake to get the bread out. Before slicing, let it cool, standing up on a rack.

108. PEAR AND CHOCOLATE GALETTE

Prep Time: 40 Minutes | Cook Time: 40 Minutes

Total Times: 1 hour 20 Minutes | Serving: 10

Ingredients

- 75g coconut oil
- 4-5 pears
- pinch of salt
- a pinch of unrefined salt
- 80g dark chocolate
- 150g buckwheat flour
- 1 tbsp tapioca
- 75g almonds or almond flour
- 50ml water

- ½ lemon
- 40g chickpea flour
- 35-45g coconut sugar
- 2 tbsp maple syrup

To brush:

- 1 tbsp maple syrup
- 1 tsp non-dairy milk

Instructions

1. Get the oven ready at 180°C.
2. Apply a food processor to blend the almonds until they look like flour.
3. Use the kneading setting on your bread machine for about 10 minutes to make the galette dough.
4. In the bread pan, put the buckwheat flour, almond flour, chickpea flour, coconut sugar, and salt. Then, take the coconut oil, which should be at room temperature or slightly warmed (it should be creamy and soft, not liquid and hot), and knead while slowly adding the 50ml of cold water.
5. Please make a ball, wrap it in plastic, and take it in the refrigerator for 15 to 20 minutes.
6. In the meantime, break up the dark chocolate into chunks.
7. Wash and dry the pears, then cut them into thin slices after removing the core and seeds.
8. The pears can be put in a bowl or spread out on a piece of parchment paper. Add the lemon juice and syrup, or brush them on. Mix it gently with your hands or a wooden spoon, and set it aside for now. Put the pastry out of the refrigerator and let it set for two to 3 minutes. Do it with your hands and roll it out between 2 pieces of parchment paper with a rolling pin. About 2 to 3 mm should be the thickness of the dough.
9. Stretch the chopped chocolate over the pastry, leaving a 3cm border around the edge.

10. Place the chopped pears on top of the chocolate. Close the tart's edges and brush the pastry with the syrup and milk mixture.
11. Bake the pastry for about 38 to 40 minutes or until it turns brown.
12. You can serve the chocolate and pear galette hot or at room temperature with chocolate that has been melted.

109.BRIOCHE BURGER BUNS

Prep Time: 10 Minutes | Cook Time: 15-20 Minutes | Rising time: 1 hour

Total Times: 1 hour 25-30 Minutes | Serving: 8-12

Ingredients

- 100g butter
- seeds
- 1 egg yolk
- 10g salt
- 2 eggs
- 60g potato starch
- 20g fresh yeast
- 250ml lukewarm milk
- 440g gluten-free bread flour
- 60g brown sugar

Instructions

1. Mix the yeast with warm milk that is about 25°C.
2. Put the yeast that has been diluted and the milk in the bread pan. Then, put the other ingredients in the order shown. Choose the setting for bread dough.
3. Take the dough out, press it down with your fist at the conclusion of the program, and divide it into six to eight equal pieces to form small rolls. Take them on a baking sheet with parchment paper, leaving enough space between each one. Warp them with a damp tea towel and let them rise for an hour, preferably in an oven with a temperature of less than 30°C.
4. Brush them with egg wash after the dough has risen, and then top them with a few seeds.
5. Set the oven on to 180°C and bake until golden brown.

110. DAIRY-FREE DINNER ROLLS

Prep Time: 15 Minutes | Cook Time: 20 Minutes

Mixing time & Rise time: 1 hour 45 Minutes | Total Times: 2 hours 45 Minutes | Serving: 24

Ingredients

- ¼ cup of sugar
- 1 Tbsp active dry yeast
- 1 tsp xanthan gum
- 45 grams of tapioca starch, about ⅓ cup of
- 1 ¼ cups of white rice flour, about 1 ¼ cups of 220 grams
- 1 tsp salt
- 120 grams potato starch, about ¾ cup of
- 1 egg
- 2 cups of water warmed to 80 F
- 1 cup of brown rice flour, about 155 grams
- ⅓ cup of dairy-free butter softened

Instructions

1. Take all the ingredients in your bread machine in the order that the manufacturer suggests. See the first note.
2. Putting liquid into the breadmaker
3. Set the machine to mix the dough.
4. The dough's consistency in the bead machine
5. Spray each cup of in 2 muffin tins with cooking spray to get them ready. Set aside.
6. Prepared muffin tins for baking rolls
7. After the dough has been mixed for a while, take the pan out of the machine.
8. The bread machine finished mixing the dough.
9. To put the batter in muffin cups of, use a large scoop or a large spoon. Half-fill each cup.
10. fill the muffin tins with batter
11. Put the pans in a warm place for 15 minutes to let the dough rise.
12. Rolls after rising.
13. Place your oven to 400 degrees F and bake for 20 minutes.
14. rolls after baking, sitting in pans
15. Get out of the pan and put on a wire rack to cool down more. Warm is best.
16. There are 24 rolls on a wire rack.

111. SOFT DINNER ROLL

Prep Time: 10 Minutes | Cook Time: 15 Minutes | Rising time: 30 minutes

Total Times: Minutes Serving: 12 rolls

Ingredients

- 3 tbsp vegetable oil
- 1 1/4 cups of water
- 3 large eggs
- 3 tbsp honey

Dry mixture:

- 1/2 cup of cornstarch
- 1 (0.25 ounce) package (7g) or 2 1/4 tsp Red Star Active Dry Yeast
- 1 tbsp xanthan gum
- 2/3 cup of tapioca flour
- 1 1/2 cups of garfava bean flour
- 1/3 cup of rice flour
- 1 1/2 tsp salt

Instructions

1. Prepare pan: Grease a muffin tin with 12 cups of and set it aside.
2. Check sure that everything is at room temperature. Pour the mixture of water, eggs, oil, and honey into a baking pan. Mix dry ingredients together well in a mixing bowl. Add to the baking pan's liquid ingredients.
3. Choose the DOUGH cycle, but stop the machine as soon as the mixing is done. Don't let the dough rise in the machine.
4. Spoon the batter into the muffin cups of that have been prepared, and let it rise for about 30 minutes.
5. Turn oven on to 375°F.
6. Until the tops are golden brown, bake for 15 minutes. Warm is best.

112. CINNAMON ROLLS

Prep Time: 10 Minutes | Cook Time: 20 Minutes | Additional Time: 35-40 Minutes

Total Times: 65-70 Minutes | Serving: 12

Ingredients
Dough:

- 1 cup of plus 2 tbsp warm milk
- 1/2 cup of sugar
- 3 tbsp oil
- 4 cups of flour
- 1 egg, lightly beaten, plus 2 egg whites
- 3 tsp yeast
- 1 tsp salt

- 2 tbsp cinnamon
- 1 cup of brown sugar
- 2 tbsp butter

Icing:

- 1/4 cup of butter
- 1/4 tsp salt
- 1 tsp vanilla
- 1 1/2 cups of confectioners sugar
- 3 ounce cream cheese

Filling:

Instructions

1. Take the dough ingredients in the bread machine in the order given, and start the dough cycle.
2. Roll the dough into a large rectangle after the dough cycle is complete; do this by dusting the work surface with flour.
3. Spread 2 tbsp of melted butter on top, then pour the brown sugar and cinnamon mixture on top of that.
4. Roll it up, cut it into 12 equal pieces, and put them in a rectangular pan or two round cake pans that have been greased. Bake it for around 20 minutes at 325 degrees or until browned.
5. Combine the cream cheese icing by whipping together cream cheese, butter, confectioners sugar, vanilla, and salt while the cinnamon rolls are baking.
6. Put the cinnamon rolls out of the oven and let them cool down for 10 to 15 minutes before you frost them.
7.

113. CINNAMON FRUIT AND SEED LOAF

Prep Time: 15 Minutes | Cook Time: 445 Minutes

Total Times: 1 Hour | Serving: 1 loaf

Ingredients

- 100 g melted unsalted butter or dairy-free spread
- 50 g mixed seeds (Example: sesame, pumpkin, sunflower)
- 1 tsp vanilla extract
- 100g dried fruit (e.g., prunes, apricots, raisins, goji berries)
- 1 tsp xanthan gum
- 150g milk (or almond milk)
- 1 tbsp ground cinnamon
- 0.5tsp sea salt
- 30 g caster sugar or honey
- 1 tsp baking powder
- 400g gluten-free bread flour
- 120g warm water
- 2beaten egg
- 15g fast-acting yeast

Instructions

1. Put the dried fruit in the warm water and let it soak for 5 to 19 minutes. This will soften the fruit. Put the fruit, water, and the rest of the ingredients into the loaf pan.
2. Stir briefly in the loaf pan to mix.
3. Put the loaf pan into the bread maker. Put the lid on.
4. Choose the "gluten-free bread" setting. Hit "start."
5. Your loaf is done when the machine beeps. Enjoy.

114. DRIED FRUITS BREAD

Prep Time: 10 Minutes | Cook Time: 40 Minutes | Proffing Time: 2 Hour 30 Minutes

Total Times: 3Hour 20 Minutes | Serving: 1 Loaf

Ingredients

- 1 tbsp ground psyllium husks
- 70g dried fruits
- 550g KOMEKO rice flour
- 1 tbsp syrup
- 1 tsp xanthan gum
- 2 tsp xylitol sugar
- 1 tsp gingerbread spice
- 2 tbsp chia seeds
- 1 packet of dry yeast
- 450ml lukewarm water
- 3 tsp cinnamon

Instructions

1. In a bowl, mix all the yeast, sugar, and 100 ml of lukewarm water until the yeast is dissolved. Then wait 5 to 10 minutes.
2. Make small pieces out of the dried fruits.
3. Mix the dry ingredients roughly with a spatula as you add them one by one to the bread pan of your Croustina.
4. Mix well with a spatula the yeast mixture, the syrup, and the rest of the warm water.
5. Close Croustina and choose program 14 to make bread that doesn't contain gluten.
6. After the time for kneading, open the lid again and, if you want, take the dough hook out of the bread pan.
7. Now, use a spatula to shape the dough in the bread pan. To do this, push the dough from the edges down and toward the middle. This will make a loaf of bread with a beautiful shape.
8. Cut the dough on the surface of the Croustina three times, and then close the lid.
9. Keep going with program 14 until the time for rising and then baking is up.
10. Take the bread pan out of your Croustina, take out the bread loaf, and let it cool down completely.

115.FRUIT LOAF

Prep Time: 10 Minutes | Cook Time: 2 hours 30 Minutes

Total Times: 2 hours 40 Minutes | Serving: 12

Ingredients

- 330g gluten-free strong white bread flour
- 1tbsp mixed spice
- 2 eggs
- 150g mixed dried fruit
- 300ml milk
- 50ml vegetable oil
- 4tbsp sugar
- 2tsp gluten-free dry yeast
- 1tsp apple cider vinegar
- 1tsp salt

Instructions

1. Mix the milk, cider vinegar, oil, and eggs in a jug, then pour the mixture into the pan of a bread maker.
2. Mix all the flour, salt, and sugar together with a sieve, and then pour them on top of the wet ingredients.
3. Sprinkle yeast and spices on top and put the lid back on.
4. The following step will depend on your breadmaker. If yours is like mine and has a dispenser for fruit and nuts, put the fruit in the dispenser, switch to a regular setting that uses rising, turn it on, and let it do its thing. If you don't have a breadmaker with a fruit and nut dispenser, put the fruit in with the yeast and spices and switch to the gluten-free bread setting or the regular bread setting if you don't have a gluten-free option. Just like that!

5. When it's done, put it out of the bread machine and cut it!

116. FRUIT BREAD

Prep Time: 10 Minutes | Cook Time: 2 Hour 30 Minutes

Total Times: 2 Hour 40 Minutes | Serving: 12 Slice

Ingredients

- 1 tbsp white sugar
- 605g gluten-free flour
- 2 ½ tbsp brown sugar
- 1 ¼ tsp ground cinnamon
- 1 tsp white vinegar
- 1 ¼ tsp salt
- 1 tbsp xanthan gum
- 100g dried fruit and nuts (We used dried apricots, dates, and walnuts)
- 60g brown rice flour
- 2 tsp dried yeast
- 440mls water
- 80mls olive oil
- 3 eggs

Instru.ctions

1. Take all of the ingredients in the pan in the order shown. Put the lid on.
2. Set the oven to "gluten-free."
3. After it's done baking, let the bread cool for 5 minutes.
4. This bread freezes well after being cut into slices. Toast to warm up.

117. FRUIT PECAN BREAD

Prep Time: 15 Minutes | Cook Time: 2 Hour 15 Minutes

Total Times: 2 Hour 30 Minutes | Serving: 1 loaf

Ingredients

- 1/2 cup of Water
- 1 Tbsp unsalted butter
- 1/4 tsp Orange Zest
- 3/4 tsp Salt
- 3/4 cup of Mixed Dried Fruit chopped
- 1-3/4 cups of Unbleached White All-Purpose Flour
- 1-1/2 tsp Bread Machine Yeast
- 1/2 cup of Pecans chopped, toasted
- 1/3 cup of Orange Juice
- 1/2 cup of Oat Bran Cereal or Organic Oat Bran Cereal
- 1 Tbsp Non-Fat Dry Milk Powder
- 1 Egg
- 1 Tbsp Sugar

Instructions

1. Use the "Sweet Bread" setting on the bread machine. Take all the dry ingredients into the bread machine's bucket, along with the water, juice, zest, egg, and butter. Set the machine to beep when more ingredients need to be added. Start machine. When the machine beeps, add the pecans and dried fruit.
2. When the food is done cooking, take it out of the machine and the bucket and take it on a wire rack to cool. Serve with cream cheese spread when it has cooled down. This will make one loaf of bread.

118. FESTIVE FRUIT BREAD

Prep Time: 30 Minutes | Cook Time: 1 Hour 50 Minutes

Total Times: 2 Hour 20 Minutes | Serving: 1 loaf

Ingredients

Wet ingredients:

- 3 large eggs
- 1/4 cup of vegetable oil
- 1 2/3 cups of water

Dry ingredients:

- 1 tsp ground nutmeg
- 1/2 cup of tapioca flour

- 1 (0.25 ounce) package (7g) or 2 1/4 tsp Red Star Active Dry Yeast
- 1 1/2 tsp salt
- 2 cups of white rice flour
- 1/2 cup of potato starch
- 3 tbsp granulated sugar
- 1 tbsp xanthan gum
- 1 (6 or 7 ounce) package of dried fruit, finely chopped
- 1/3 cup of cornstarch

Instructions

1. Check sure that everything is at room temperature. Take the wet ingredients in a bowl with a whisk, then put the mixture into a baking pan. Take all the dry ingredients in a separate bowl and whisk them together. Then, Take the dry ingredients on top of the wet ingredients in the baking pan.
2. Choose the gluten-free cycle and turn on the machine. After the mixing starts, use a rubber spatula to work any unmixed ingredients into the dough. Stay near the edges and top of the batter to keep the kneading blade from getting in the way.
3. Take the pan out of the machine when the cycle is done, then the bread stays in the pan for around ten minutes, then flip the pan over and provide it a gentle shake to get the bread out. Before slicing, let it cool, standing up on a rack.

119. CARDAMOM FLAVORED FRUIT BREAD

Prep Time: 2 Hour 45 Minutes | Cook Time: 30 Minutes

Total Times: 3 Hour 15 Minutes | Serving: 1 loaf

Ingredients
Wet ingredients:

- 4 tbsp vegetable oil
- 1 2/3 cups of water
- 1 tsp cider vinegar
- 3 large eggs

Dry ingredients:

- 1/2 cup of dry milk powder

- 2/3 cup of potato starch
- 2 tsp ground cardamom
- 3 tbsp granulated sugar
- 2 1/2 tsp xanthan gum
- 6 ounces package of dried fruit bits
- 1 (0.25 ounce) package (7g) or 2 1/4 tsp Red Star Active Dry Yeast
- 1 1/2 tsp salt
- 1/3 cup of tapioca flour
- 2 cups of white rice flour

Instructions

1. Check sure that everything is at room temperature. Take the wet ingredients in a bowl with a whisk, then put the mixture into a baking pan. Take all the dry ingredients in a separate bowl and whisk them together. Then, Take the dry ingredients on top of the wet ingredients in the baking pan.
2. Choose the gluten-free cycle and turn on the machine. After the mixing starts, use a rubber spatula to work any unmixed ingredients into the dough. Stay near the edges and top of the batter to keep the kneading blade from getting in the way.
3. Take the pan out of the machine when the cycle is done, then the bread stays in the pan for around ten minutes, then flip the pan over and provide it a gentle shake to get the bread out. Before slicing, let it cool, standing up on a rack.

120. TOASTED OAT FRUIT BREAD

Prep Time: 20 Minutes | Cook Time: 1 hour 40 Minutes

Total Times: 2 hours | Serving: 1

Ingredients

- ¼ cup of (50g) sugar
- 1 cup of dried fruit-cranberries/and blueberries
- ¾ cup of (150g) unsweetened applesauce
- ¼ cup of (56g) vegetable or coconut oil
- ½ tsp sugar (for proofing yeast- not needed for bread machine recipe)
- 10 ounce warm water (260-280g)
- 470 g Montana Gluten Free All Purpose Baking Mix

Instructions

1. Mix applesauce, water, oil, and sugar together in a bowl, then put the mixture into the bread machine.
2. Add baking mix for all purposes and dried fruit to the machine.
3. On top of the other elements, sprinkle the yeast.
4. Start the bread machine.
5. During the mixing cycle, use a rubber spatula to make sure that no dried mixture is left on the sides or in the corners.
6. At the start of the rising time, take the mixing paddle out and smooth out the dough.
7. The recipe makes a 1.5-pound loaf of bread.

121. RIPE BANANA BREAD

Prep Time: 20 Minutes | Cook Time: 1 hour 20 Minutes

Total Times: 1 hour 20 Minutes | Serving: 12 slices

Ingredients

- 8 Tbsp – Unsalted Butter (softened) – 115 grams
- 1 Tsp – Baking Soda – 5 grams
- 2 – Large Eggs
- 2 Cups of – Gluten Free All Purpose Flour (320 grams)
- 1 Tsp – Baking Powder – 4 grams
- 1 Tsp – Vanilla Extract – 5 milliliters
- 1/2 Tsp – Salt – 3 grams
- 1 1/4 Cups of – Bananas (ripe) – 288 grams – Roughly 2 1/2 large bananas
- 1 Cup of Light Brown Sugar (packed cup of) (215 grams)
- 1/2 cup of MINI chocolate chips (67 grams) or 1/2 Cup of Chopped Walnuts (58 grams) Optional

Instructions

1. About 1:40 hours is the total machine time. FYI, the machine will mix for about 20 minutes and bake for about 1:20 hours.
2. Settings for a bread machine: Cake/Quick Bread, Light Color, 2 pound
3. Beat the eggs just a little.
4. Use a fork to mash the bananas.
5. Use your microwave to melt the butter.
6. Turn off your bread machine and take the bread pan out of it.
7. Add the bananas that have been mashed, the butter, and the eggs to the bread pan. Then add the other ingredients. Try to put the ingredients in the bread pan in the order shown above, with the wet ingredients going in first and the dry ingredients going in second. FYI: Please read the "premixing" note below before putting the ingredients in the bread pan. Also, you don't add chopped nuts or chocolate chips, which are optional at this point. They come afterward.

122. BREAD WITH SUNDRIED TOMATOES AND PARMESAN

Prep Time: 15 Minutes | Cook Time: 1 hour 45 Minutes

Total Times: 2 hours | Serving: 80-12

Ingredients

- 1tspSalt
- 2tspYeast
- 50gChopped Sundried Tomatoes
- 50gGrated Parmesan Cheese
- 1tspSugar
- 4tspVegetable Oil
- 1tspCider Vinegar
- 450gGluten-free Flour
- 320mlWater
- 1Medium Egg
- 1Medium Egg White

Instructions

1. In a mixing bowl, pour water.
2. Add vegetable oil to the bowl.
3. Crack a medium-sized egg into the bowl.
4. Add the egg white of another medium-sized egg to the bowl.
5. Gradually incorporate the gluten-free flour into the mixture.
6. Sprinkle salt and sugar into the bowl.
7. Add grated Parmesan cheese and chopped sun-dried tomatoes.
8. Sprinkle yeast over the ingredients in the bowl.
9. Set the bread machine to program 14, ensuring the crust setting is dark.

Made in the USA
Columbia, SC
25 September 2023

23369960R00078